Sports Injuries in Children and Adolescents

Rosa Mónica Rodrigo • Joan C. Vilanova
José Martel

Sports Injuries in Children and Adolescents

A Case-Based Approach

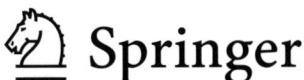

Rosa Mónica Rodrigo
Radiology Department
Resonancia Magnetica Bilbao S.A
Bilbao
Spain

José Martel
Department of Radiology
Hospital Universitario Fundación Alcorcón
Madrid
Spain

Joan C. Vilanova
Department of Radiology
Clínica Girona-Hospital
Sta.Caterina University of Girona
Girona
Spain

ISBN 978-3-642-54745-4   ISBN 978-3-642-54746-1   (eBook)
DOI 10.1007/978-3-642-54746-1
Springer Heidelberg New York Dordrecht London

Library of Congress Control Number: 2014941945

Printed on acid-free paper

Springer is part of Springer Science+Business Media (www.springer.com)

Contents

Head and Spine Trauma

Miguel Ángel López-Pino, Elena García-Esparza,
and Javier Telletxea-Elorriaga

Contents

M.Á. López-Pino (✉) • E. García-Esparza
Department of Radiology,
Hospital Universitario "Niño Jesús", Madrid, Spain
e-mail: malopezpino@gmail.com

J. Telletxea-Elorriaga
Department of Bome Clinic, International SOS,
Bome Clinic, Bata, Equatorial Guinea

R.M. Rodrigo et al., *Sports Injuries in Children and Adolescents*,
DOI 10.1007/978-3-642-54746-1_1, © Springer-Verlag Berlin Heidelberg 2014

Case 1.1: Cervical Fracture with Spinal Lesion

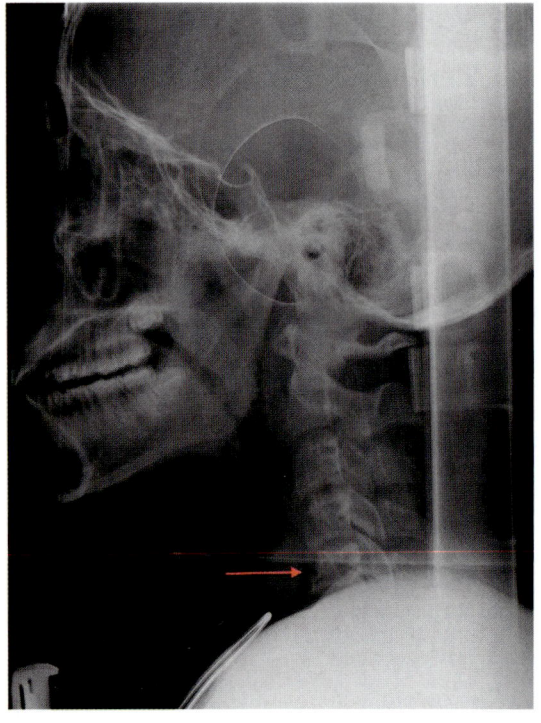

Fig. 1.1

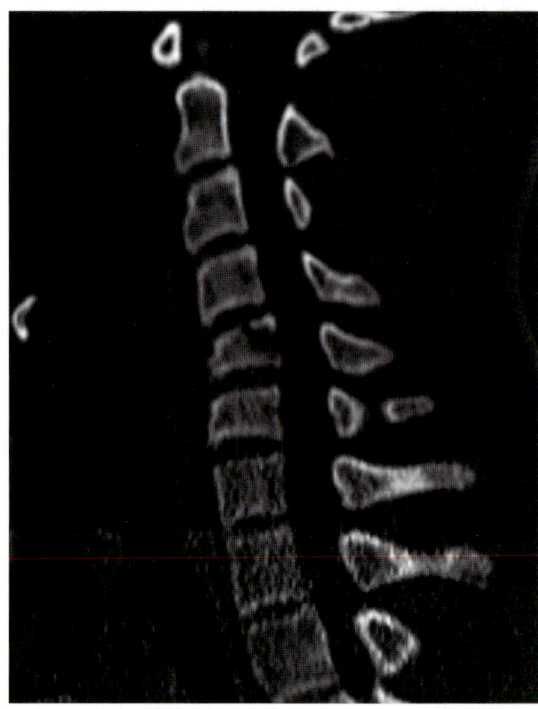

Fig. 1.2

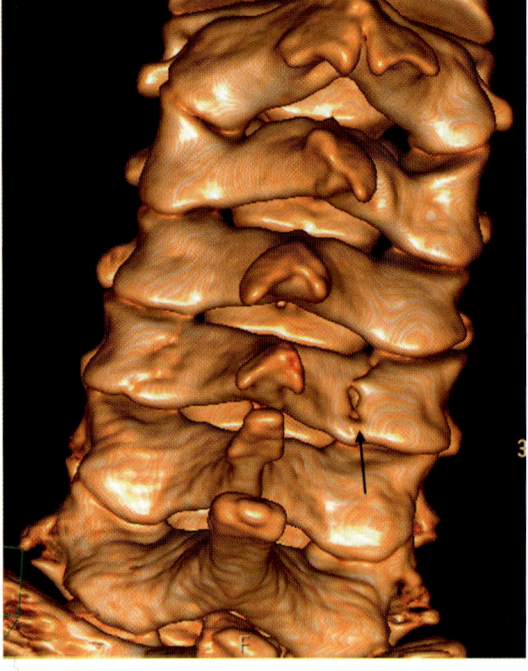

Fig. 1.3

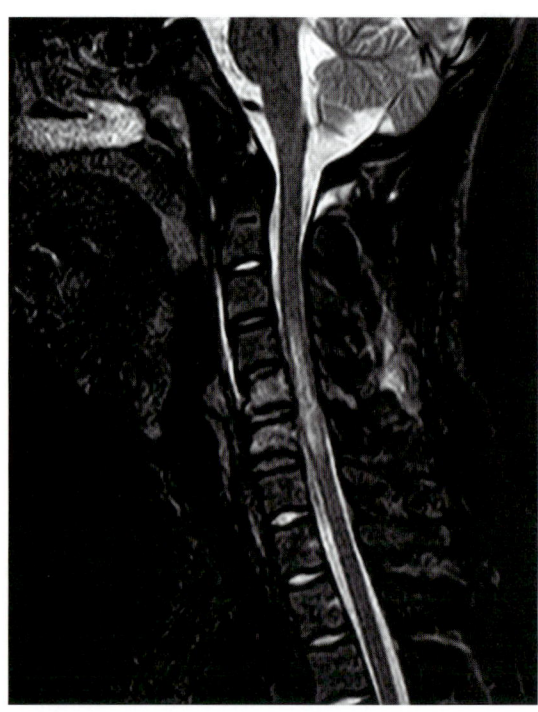

Fig. 1.4

A 16-year-old male sustains an impact with a hyperflexion cervical injury while performing a somersault during a physical education class. He presents with severe pain and power loss in both lower extremities. The paraplegia is obvious in the emergency room: muscle weakness, loss of sensation, deep tendon hyperreflexia, and autonomic function alteration, all compatible with a spinal cord lesion.

Comments

In young children, due to their biomechanical setup leading to greater flexibility (skeletal immaturity plus increased laxity in paravertebral ligaments and muscles), cervical trauma tends to occur at higher levels, from the base of the cranium to C3. The greater spine flexibility relative to the cord explains the tendency for cord damage without bony lesions. In older children and teenagers, cord injuries are more frequently seen at C5–C6 level, just like in adults.

Specific facts to be considered in pediatric cervical trauma:

- C2–C3 subluxation is physiological.
- The atlantoaxoid distance is greater than in adults.
- Odontoid fractures tend to affect the basal synchondrosis.

In a pediatric sporting activity context, cervical spine fractures with associated cord damage are typical in diving during water sports, to the point of, according to some series, being the most frequent cause for cord injury in this age group. Diving into shallow waters is particularly dangerous. In gymnastics, the mechanism of injury tends to be extreme hyperflexion with or without associated trauma.

Cervical spine radiographs, including lateral views up to C7/T1, are usually the initial diagnostic tool. However, the false negative rate with a single lateral study can reach between 21 and 26 %, so taking the clinical findings into consideration; CT should be considered to complete the exam.

CT with multiplane reformatting plays a fundamental role in cervical trauma diagnosis: it adequately shows fracture trajectories and extension in a better way than MRI.

MRI is useful in spinal cord evaluation, detecting cord lesion (with or without associated bony fracture) and possible cord compression. It is also valuable to assess the extradural space and spinal ligaments.

Radiological Findings

The plain lateral view (Fig.1.1) shows a vertebral body fracture in C5 (arrow). Given the clinical and radiological findings and the incomplete study (no views of the lower spine), a CT was performed.

A cervicothoracic CT with multiplanar reformatting in the sagittal plane (Fig. 1.2) shows C5 with an anteroposterior fracture line in the upper cortex following a right inferolateral trajectory in the anterior region of the lower cortex. The fracture line reaches the posterior wall.

The volumetric 3D reconstruction (Fig. 1.3), posterior view, shows fracture lines in both C5 laminae, with greater displacement on the right (arrow) but without interapophyseal joint disruption.

The MRI study (sagittal plane, STIR) (Fig. 1.4) shows an increased cord signal from C4 to C6 consistent with contusion. There are signal changes in C5 and C6 vertebral bodies compatible with bony edema. There is extensive soft tissue signal alteration consistent with acute posttraumatic edema.

Case 1.2: Lumbar Spondylolysis

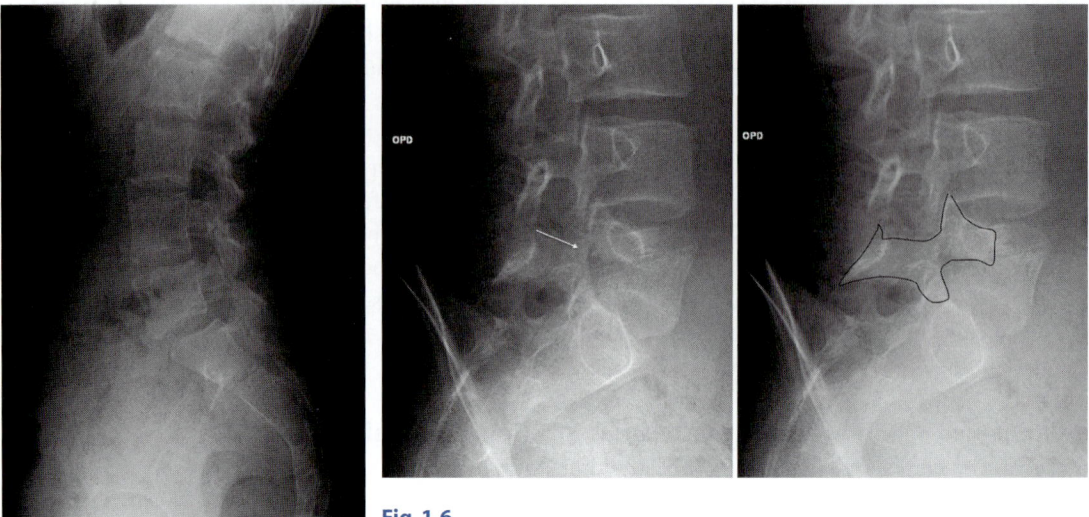

Fig. 1.6

Fig. 1.5

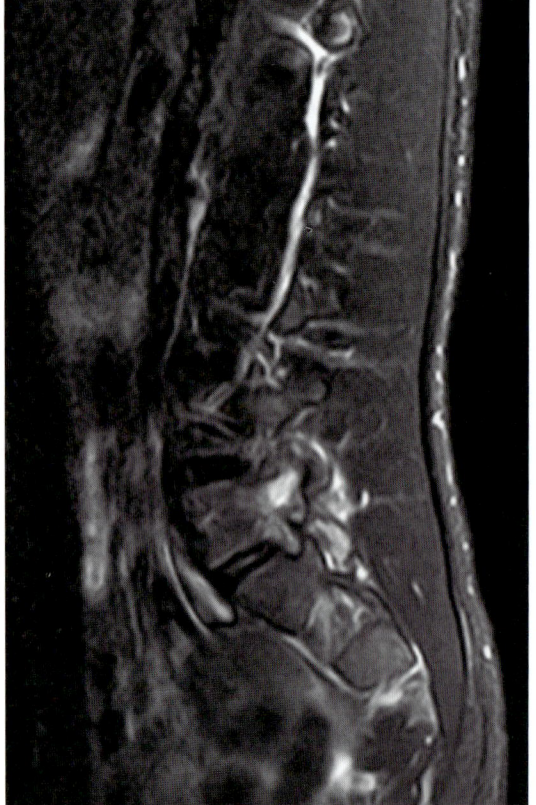

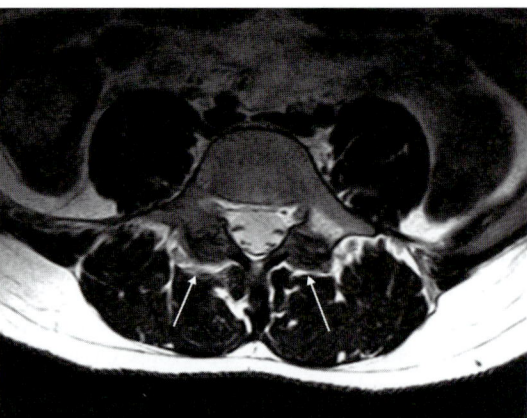

Fig. 1.8

Fig. 1.7

A 15-year-old male presented with lumbar pain for the previous 2 months, partially resolved with nonsteroidal anti-inflammatory drugs. He was a keen skate-park boarder and referred multiple trauma events although he did not recall any of them as precipitant to the presenting complaint.

Comments

Spondylolysis is fairly frequent in sporting children and teenagers. It occurs in almost half the cases consulting for lumbar pain. It can happen both with repetitive and acute trauma, mostly when subjected to flexion and hyperextension forces. It is typical in soccer players, gymnasts, swimmers, and pool divers.

It originates on a pars articularis defect on the vertebral posterior elements.

Although it can affect any level, it tends to involve L5 85–95 % of the times (the rest is mostly L4). It can be uni- or bilateral. When unilateral, a compensatory contralateral sclerosis can be seen; it should not be mistaken for other pathologies such as osteoid osteoma.

Plain lumbar spine radiographs in four views (anteroposterior, lateral, and both obliques) are required. Oblique views are needed since up to 20 % of cases are only seen in them. Interruption of LaChapelle's or Scotty dog's neck is the classical sign. A lateral radiograph may show an associated spondylolisthesis.

Given the high incidence in young sportswomen and men, if the plain radiographs are normal but the suspicion index is high, other diagnostic tools (bone scan, CT, or MRI) that could additionally detect other pathologies such as infection or osteoid sarcoma should be used.

MRI is able to determine early edema before a complete defect occurs (allowing a better response to conservative treatment). The lack of ionizing radiation for MRI makes the technique of choice to evaluate spondylolysis.

Radiological Findings

The lateral radiograph shows a normal vertebral alignment, without L5 spondylolisthesis (anterior displacement) (Fig. 1.5). It is in the oblique views (Fig. 1.6) where the pars articularis defect is noted as a fracture line (arrow) in LaChapelle's dog's neck.

MRI proved relevant edema both in the pars and in the pedicles as seen in sagittal STIR (Fig. 1.7) and T2-weighted axial views (Fig. 1.8). Also, the bilateral spondylolysis can be appreciated as a bilateral defect in L5's pars interarticularis (arrow) in the axial views.

Case 1.3: Isolated Spinous Process Fracture

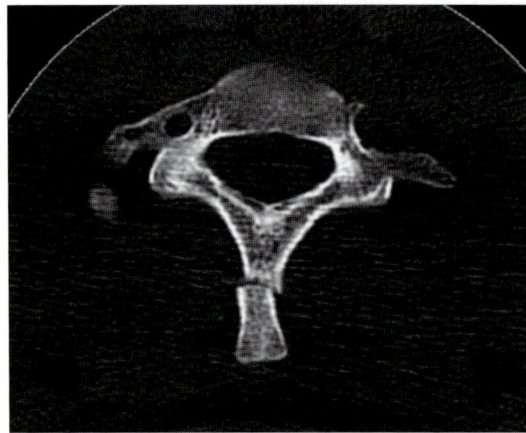

Fig. 1.9

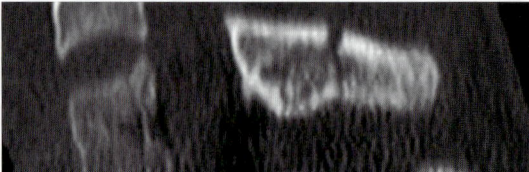

Fig. 1.10

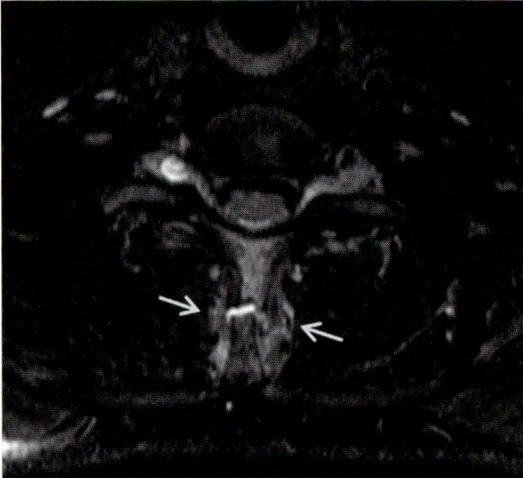

Fig. 1.11

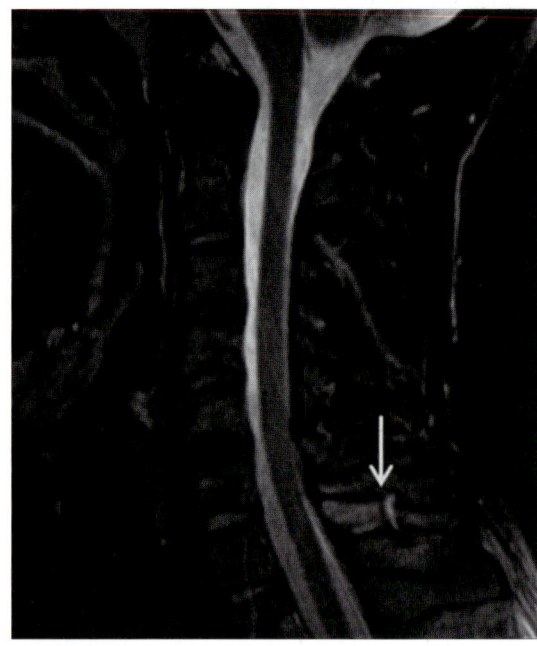

Fig. 1.12

A 16-year-old soccer player got injured after forcibly hyperextending his neck trying to head the ball towards another player. He presented with pain and decreased range of cervical flexion–extension. There was pain on palpation of the lower cervical spinous processes.

Comment

Isolated spinous process fractures (Clay-shoveler fracture) are fairly infrequent, and they are generally considered stable. However, they can also be associated to more significant lesions depending on the forces involved.

They were first described in Western Australia among strenuous physical laborers. They have been reported in American football, volleyball, power lifting, golf, cycling, diving, skiing, ice hockey, wrestling, and gymnastics and, anecdotally, among Nintendo Wii players and indoor rock climbers.

They usually occur at lower cervical/ upper thoracic levels. Mechanisms of injury include hyperflexion, hyperextension, rotation, or repetitive stress. In these cases the para- and supraspinous musculature and ligaments can avulse the spinous process. When caused by a direct blow, they may be associated to other more serious injuries or extend into the laminar regions. In high-risk incidents, exquisite care should be taken to rule out unstable injuries capable of spinal cord or nerve root damage.

Plain radiography (AP, lateral, and odontoid views) constitutes the initial investigation of choice. A ghost sign, where a double spinous process is seen on the AP view, results from displacement of the fracture.

Patients with associated injuries *or* presenting after a high-risk mechanism of injury *or* those showing radiological abnormalities on initial studies require CT investigation with coronal and sagittal reformatted views.

MRI is useful in investigating suspected muscular, ligamentous, and spinal cord injuries. CT and/or MR angiogram are required to discard vascular injuries.

Isolated spinous process fractures are almost always managed conservatively with rest, analgesia, and immobilization during the painful period followed in due course by physical therapy. They may become chronically symptomatic in particular if nonunion is present.

Our player's management included soft collar immobilization for 10 days. Jogging was introduced on day 15 post injury and more complex football drills on his own at day 40. He was discharged back to full training at day 72.

Radiological Findings

The axial (Fig. 1.9) and sagittal reconstruction CT (Fig. 1.10) show the C7 spinous process fracture.

The axial fat-suppressed FSE T2-weighted MR image (Fig. 1.11) shows the fracture and surrounding edema (arrows).

The sagittal fat-suppressed FSE T2-weighted MR image (Fig. 1.12) shows the fracture with no other acute injury related.

Case 1.4: Cranial Fracture with Intraparenchymal Contusion/Hematoma

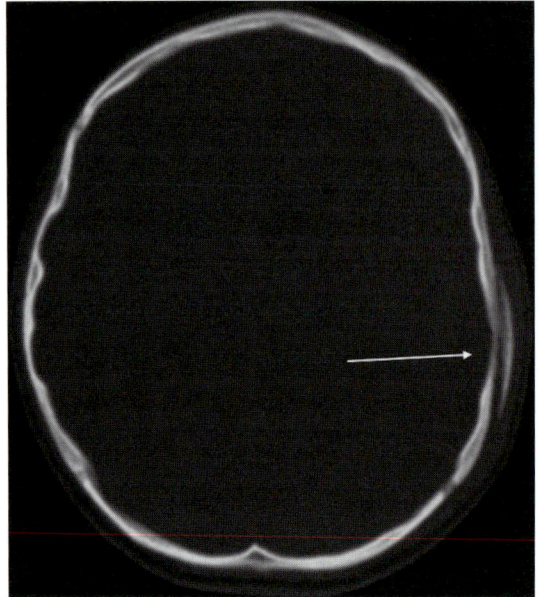

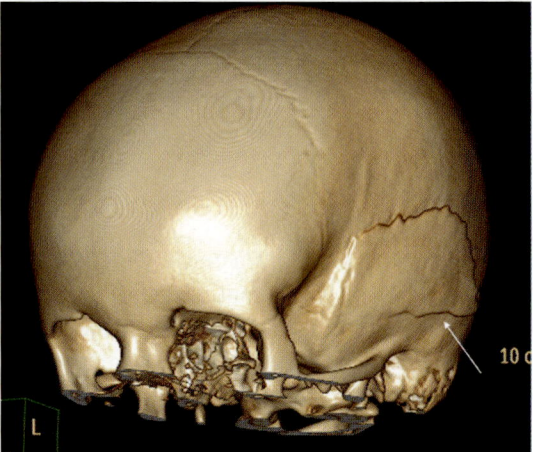

Fig. 1.14

Fig. 1.13

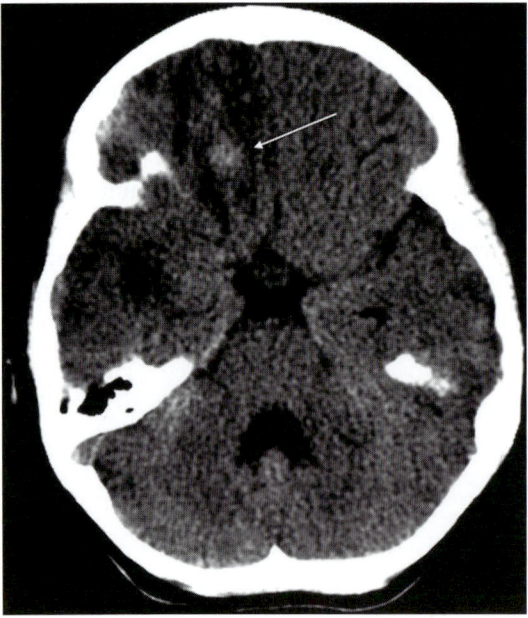

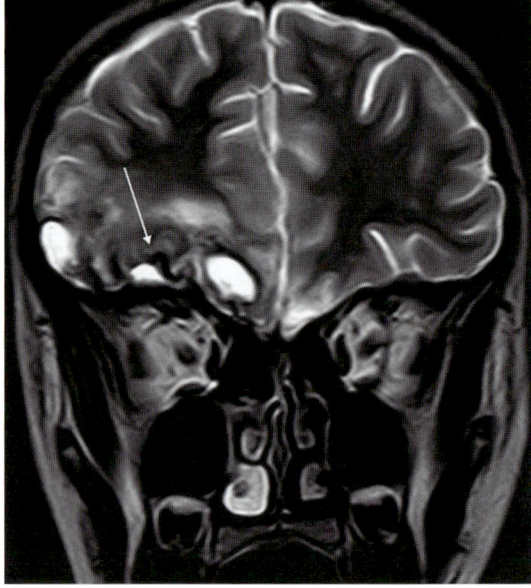

Fig. 1.15

Fig. 1.16

A 13-year-old male suffered a head injury after a cycling accident. He was brought to the emergency room with temporary loss of consciousness and severe headache. On examination, there was an obvious cranial nerve VI lesion on the right side.

Comment

Cycling accidents are the most common cause of head injury in older children and teenagers. While most of them are mild, detecting intracranial lesions requiring extended management is paramount. The choice of diagnostic imaging techniques is dictated by clinical findings and evaluation including a Glasgow Coma Scale.

Contrary to adults, in smaller children, due to the head's larger relative volume and the skull's increased flexibility and fragility, a lower energy impact can lead to skull fractures. Plain radiography can detect most of them (seen as radiolucent linear images). A fracture increases the chances of intracranial lesions, but its absence does not exclude significant parenchymal damage, so plain radiography is not useful as a screening tool. Over 50 % cases combine intracranial lesions with normal plain radiographs, and about half detected skull fractures are associated to intraparenchymal injury.

CT's speed and ability to detect acute traumatic lesions make it the investigation of choice to diagnose and follow up pediatric head injuries. If the fracture is parallel to axial cuts, multiplane 3D reconstructions or MIP (Maximum Intensity Projection) may be required.

Intra-axial lesions are mostly constituted by contusions, intraparenchymal hematomas, and shearing lesions.

In children, the greater cranial flexibility increases the risk for intraparenchymal damage. This can be caused by either direct trauma or secondary to acceleration–deceleration mechanisms. Their main locations are as follows: temporal lobe (temporal pole, inferior temporal region and adjacent to the Sylvian fisure), frontal lobe, frontal lobe (inferior frontal region), and parasagittal areas.

Contusions are seen in CT as poorly defined, low-density areas. Hyperdense foci can be noted in superficial gray matter if hemorrhage is present.

MRI has a greater sensitivity in detecting non-hemorrhagic contusions: FLAIR sequence on MRI shows cortical edema, while T2 echo-gradient sequence detects chronic hemorrhage and hemosiderin deposits.

Radiological Findings

Helicoidal CT without contrast shows a left temporal fracture (arrow) with overlapping on the bony window (Fig. 1.13). A volumetric 3D reconstruction is performed to better appreciate the whole fracture (arrow) (Fig. 1.14). The parenchymal window (Fig. 1.15) shows hemorrhagic contusions (highly attenuated foci) in right basal frontal (arrow) and anterior temporal regions with perilesional vasogenic edema.

MRI: a cortex/subcortex fuzzy lesion, mostly hyperintense, with decreased signal in relation to hemosiderin (arrow) in the right anterior frontal and temporal regions compatible with evolving trauma is noted on the T2-weighted coronal plane (Fig. 1.16).

Case 1.5: Cranial Fracture with Epidural Hematoma

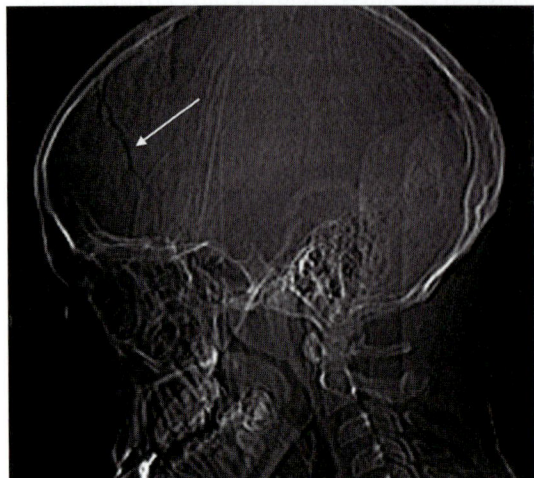

Fig. 1.17

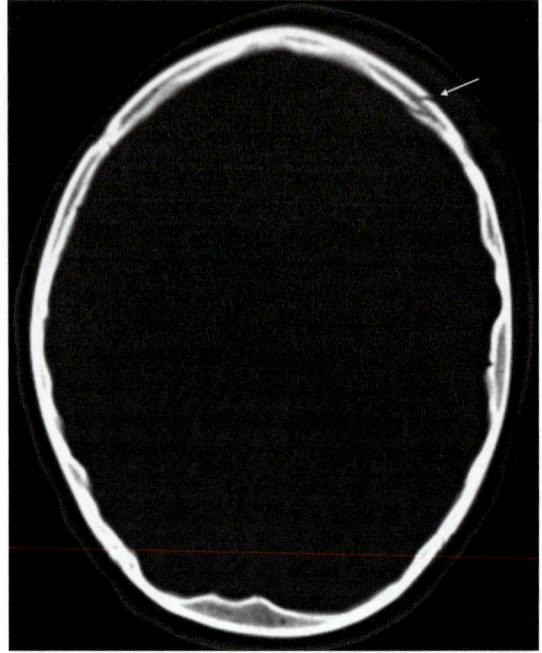

Fig. 1.18

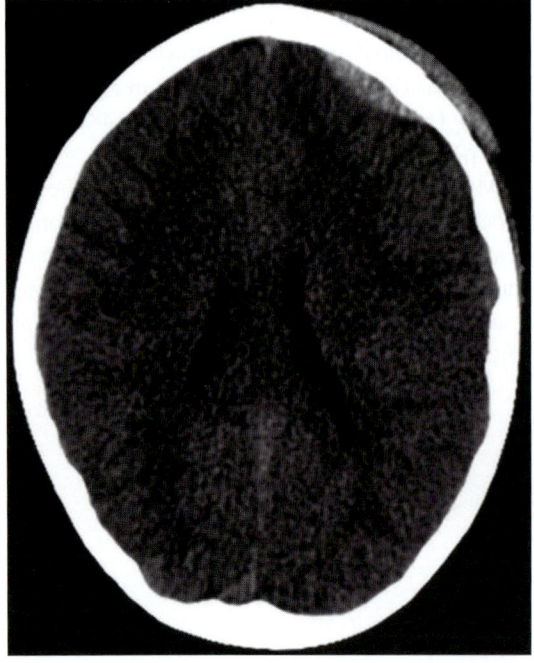

Fig. 1.19

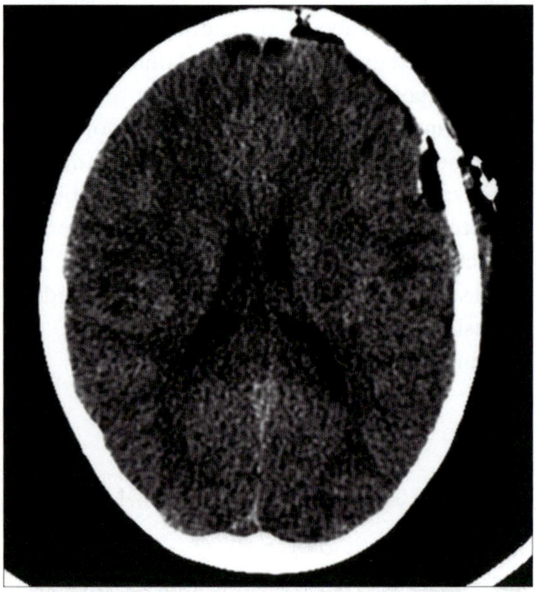

Fig. 1.20

A 9-year-old boy suffered a frontal head trauma following a goal frame falling on him. After a lucid interval he presented with headache and deteriorating conscious level.

Comments

Head trauma during soccer practice is more common among the 10–14 age group. The main mechanism of injury tends to involve a direct collision with another player, specifically, head to head. In the 5–9-year-old age group, there is a high proportion of head trauma caused by goal post-impact.

In addition to intraparenchymal damage, cranial trauma can be associated to extra-axial blood collection, both epidural and/or subdural.

A posttraumatic epidural hematoma is a blood collection between the dura mater and the internal skull table. It is most usually located in the temporoparietal region. It occurs in 1–3 % of moderate to severe head trauma in children.

It can have a rapid evolution, especially if arterial in origin (medial meningeal artery), thus requiring urgent diagnosis and treatment. Avoiding delays in CT evaluation is paramount. Periodic CT evaluation is also required in conservative management.

As opposed to adults, epidural hematomas in children are:
- Generally of venous origin since the medial meningeal artery's increased relative laxity decreases its injury probability. For this same reason, hematoma's growth will be slower.
- Less frequently associated to skull fractures.

CT is the investigation of choice to evaluate extra-axial (including epidural) hematomas. Its high availability in emergency departments and high sensitivity for detecting hematic collections make it extremely useful. Venous contrast is not generally employed.

Acute epidural hematomas are seen as high-density images with a typical biconvex morphology. In contrast to subdural hematomas, they do not cross over sutures but can traverse the midline.

In MRI, the signal's intensity will change with time. Its main indication in this case is in discarding intracranial and diffuse axonal injuries.

Radiological Findings

An urgent helicoidal CT without intravenous contrast was the initial imaging technique employed in this case. Plain skull radiographs are not indicated.

A frontal fracture line (arrow) is evident in the localizing image (Fig. 1.17).

The bony window in the cranial CT (Fig. 1.18) shows a left frontal fracture (arrow) secondary to direct trauma. A left frontal, extra-axial hyperdense collection with the classic biconvex shape, causing moderate mass effect against the cortical grooves, is seen in the parenchymal window (Fig. 1.19). It is situated at the fracture/encephalic hematoma site.

The hematoma progression and clinical deterioration indicated surgical drainage. Hematoma resolution with minimal postsurgical pneumocephalus is observed in the postoperative CT (Fig. 1.20)

Case 1.6: Subarachnoid Hemorrhage (SAH)

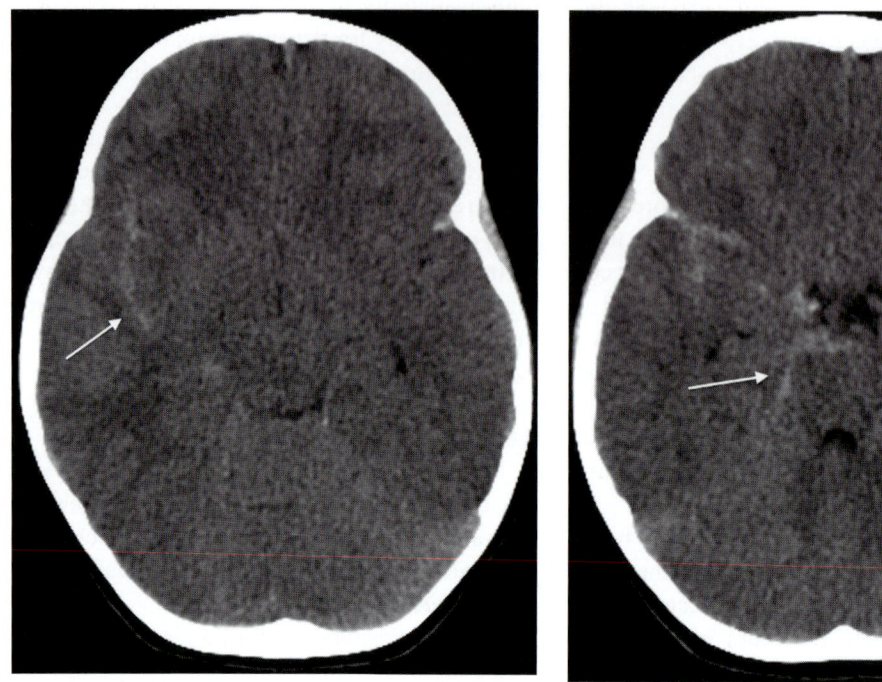

Fig. 1.21

Fig. 1.22

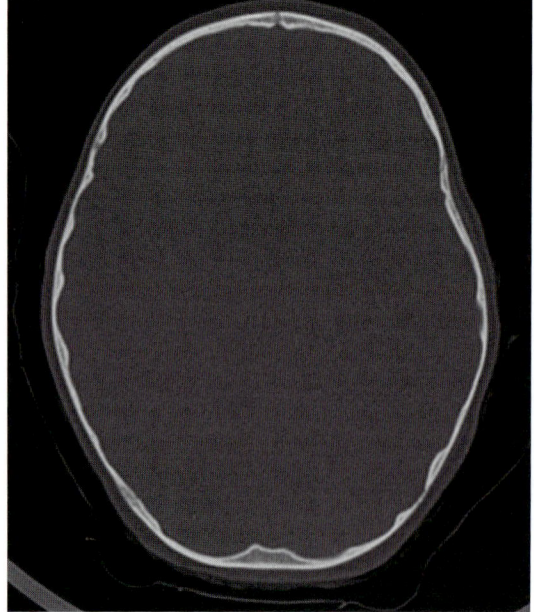

Fig. 1.23

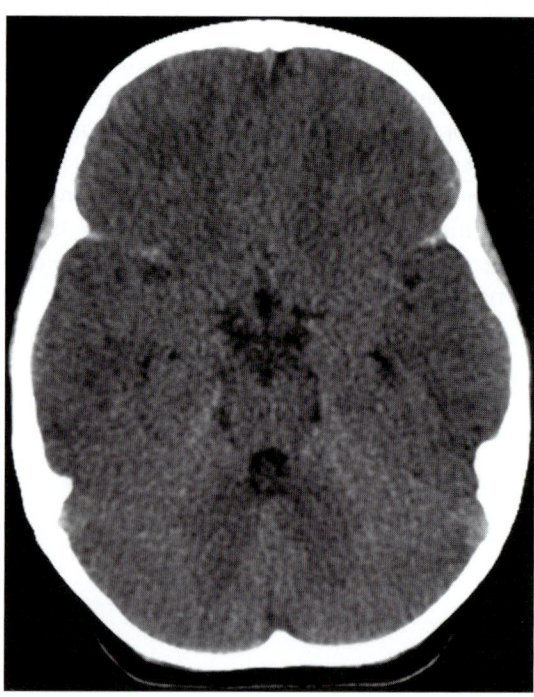

Fig. 1.24

A 6-year-old girl hit her head after falling from a horse. She was wearing protective headgear. She attended the hospital with headache and vomiting. On arrival to the ER, she presented a normal conscious level with no focal neurological deficit.

Comment

Falling while horse riding is a significant cause of injury. Although only 18 % of these are head injuries, they are the leading cause for hospital admission in this recreational activity. Wearing a hard hat can somehow decrease but not eliminate their severity.

Subarachnoid hemorrhages (SAHs) are frequently seen in moderate and severe head injuries. CT is the initial investigation of choice since it is fast and readily available in emergency room environments. Its sensitivity reaches 90 % in detecting acute subarachnoid events.

Subarachnoid hemorrhages are seen as fine hyperdense collections around the gyri of the convexity, interhemispheric sulcus and interpeduncular cistern. For those caused by trauma, the largest amount of blood tends to pool in the impact zone (generally, the brain convexity).

The FLAIR sequence on MRI is the most sensitive to detect SAH. It is seen as an extraparenchymal, hyperintense collection as opposed to the low-intensity signal generated by cerebrospinal fluid. The new susceptibility-weighted imaging (SWI) also has great sensitivity in detecting subarachnoid blood.

SAH patients should be closely monitored since vasospasm is one of their most serious complications.

Negative outcome predictors include the size of the hemorrhage, associated lesions, and decreased conscious level on hospital admission.

Radiology Findings

A cranial CT with bony reconstruction was carried out. It showed a fairly extensive SAH, particularly around the right Sylvian fissure (arrow) and adjacent gyri (Fig. 1.21), but also extending into the interpeduncular cistern (arrow) (Fig. 1.22). No associated lesions or cranial fractures were detected (Fig. 1.23).

The patient was admitted for observation and had a satisfactory evolution with good pain control and no new neurological signs.

Repeated CT 2 days later shows an almost completely resolved hemorrhage with a minimal residue along the right Sylvain fissure (Fig. 1.24).

Given the positive clinical and radiological evolution, no brain MRI was carried out.

Case 1.7: Petrous Bone Fracture

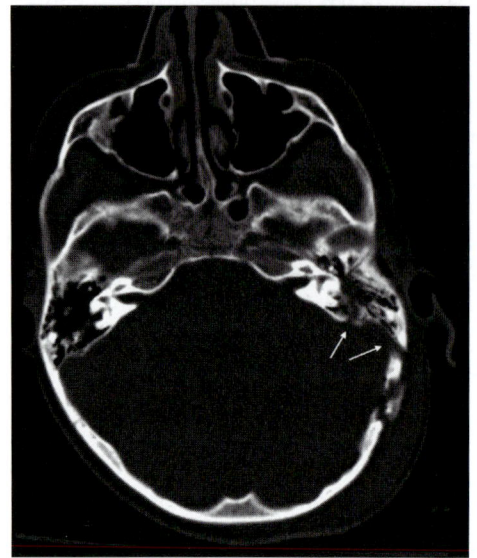

Fig. 1.25

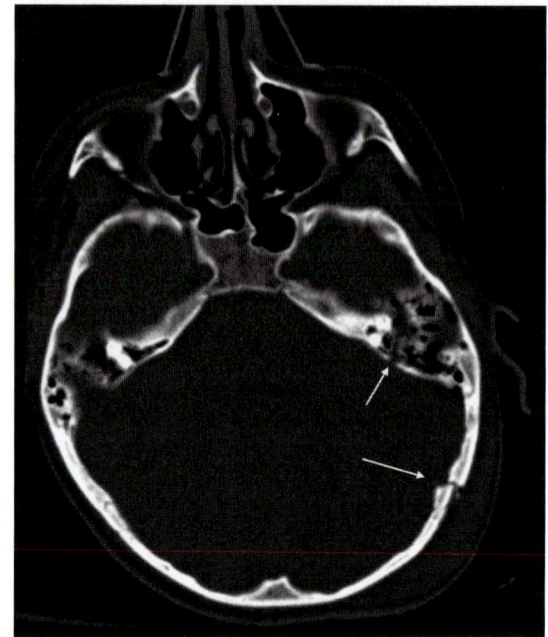

Fig. 1.26

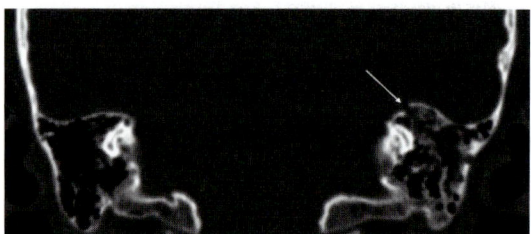

Fig. 1.27

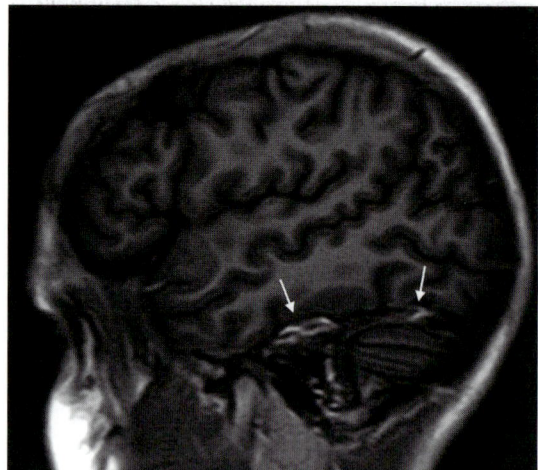

Fig. 1.28

An 11-year-old girl without protective headgear fell on the ground and hit her head while skating. She presented with moderate otorrhea on her left side.

Comment

Sport-derived craniofacial injuries are common in cycling, soccer, hockey, horse riding, skiing, skating, and baseball. The epidemiology varies depending on sport, country, and age group. They are normally caused by direct trauma (head to head, fall or strike by a sporting implement such as a baseball bat).

Multiplanar and volumetric CT is particularly useful in these cases. In petrous bone fractures, an axial high resolution or a helical sequence that would allow axial image acquisition with coronal reconstruction can be employed. Direct coronal slices are generally not possible in an acute pediatric trauma context. Deciding which technique to use would depend on the type of CT scanner available.

Petrous bone fractures can be suspected in patients with direct trauma to the temporoparietal region presenting with otorrhea or hemotympanum. It is the most frequent of all basal skull fractures. They can be associated to loss of hearing (sensorineural or transmission related) and facial nerve damage; however, they can debut with very few symptoms and can frequently be incidental CT findings.

Petrous fractures are better identified on axial CT slices. They are classified in two basic types but can present with "mixed" or oblique trajectories:

- Longitudinal fracture: parallel to the petrous temporal bone's long axis. It is the most common. They are extra-labyrinth. Facial nerve damage can occur but less frequently than in transverse fractures. There is a "posterior" subtype reflecting mastoid involvement.
- Transverse fracture: perpendicular to the petrous bone's long axis. It often reaches the internal auditory canal and the otic capsule. Facial nerve damage is more frequent, but extension into the middle ear or external auditory canal is less common.

Care must be taken to ascertain the continuity of the ossicular chain via CT, particularly to exclude incus/stapes disruption.

MRI can be useful if intracranial complications or associated pathology (posttraumatic cephalocele or intracranial hemorrhage) is suspected. Hemotympanum-related changes can also be appreciated. Facial nerve damage can usually be detected after intravenous contrast use.

Radiological Findings

Helical CT axial slices show a mixed oblique (longitudinal and transverse) fracture of the left petrous bone (Fig. 1.25) reaching the middle ear (arrow) without ossicular chain disruption. It does not affect the internal auditory canal. There is partial occupation of mastoid cells. It extends into the left parieto-occipital region (Fig. 1.26) (arrow).

The left petrous bone fracture reaching the left mastoid antrum (arrow) is seen in the coronal multiplanar reconstruction (Fig. 1.27).

The sagital MRI view on the T1 weighted image (Fig. 1.28) shows hyperintense T1 signal changes due to blood remaining within the mastoid cells/middle ear (arrow), as well as minimal extra-axial laminar bleeding adjacent to the tentorium (arrow).

Case 1.8: Mandibular Fracture

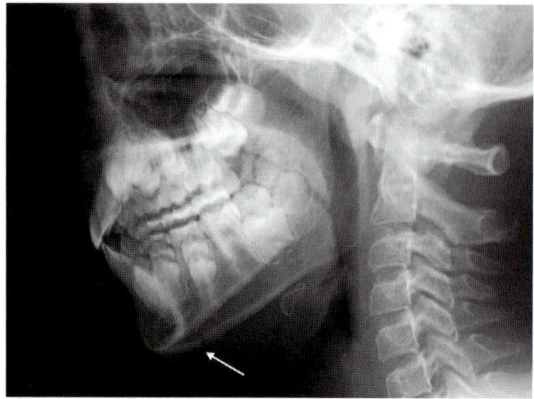

Fig. 1.29

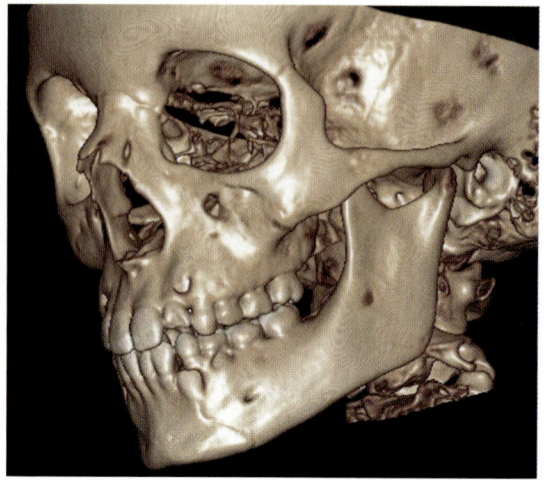

Fig. 1.30

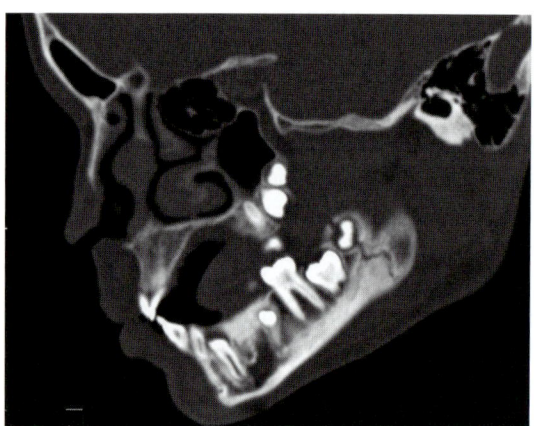

Fig. 1.31

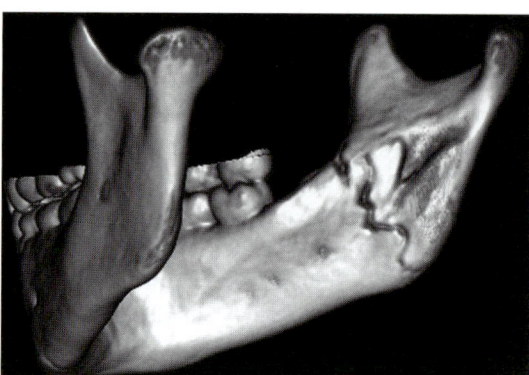

Fig. 1.32

An 11-year-old boy fell onto his jaw while high-speed skiing and was attended on the ER with severe pain and trismus.

Comment

Facial fractures are less common in children than in adults due to several different factors such as decreased paranasal sinuses pneumatization, greater bone flexibility, and lack of certain typical risk factors (occupational).

Pediatric mandibular fractures are relatively infrequent and require a substantial force. The most frequent causes are motor vehicle accidents followed by high-velocity sporting injuries (mainly cycling and falls from height). They are often associated to upper facial and cranial fractures. Areas most frequently affected are around the condyles, incisive region, and near the mandibular angle.

Plain facial region radiographs are difficult to interpret due to the complex anatomy and structure overlap. They may not show the fracture or its complete extension. If the suspicion index is high, volumetric, multiplanar CT appears as the imaging investigation of choice.

Facial fracture management in children can be controversial. Surgical fixation may alter the development of the bone and may cause an altered, uneven bite or damaged dental roots/ teeth buds.

Radiology Findings

A fracture line can be seen on the anterior mandibular region (arrow) on the lateral skull radiograph (Fig. 1.29). A CT is performed to ascertain its trajectory, to evaluate stability and analyze surgical criteria. The volumetric reconstruction (Fig. 1.30) shows a greenstick fracture on the external cortex to the left of the mandibular symphysis extending towards the un-budded incisive bed. Additionally, another greenstick fracture on the internal cortex can also be seen affecting the right mandible and extending into the last molar bed (Figs. 1.31 and 1.32).

Mandibular nerve damage and neck or condyle fractures were excluded and temporomandibular joint congruence was good.

Because of the bilateral fractures, surgical fixation was carried out despite both of them being stable.

Case 1.9: Nasal Fracture

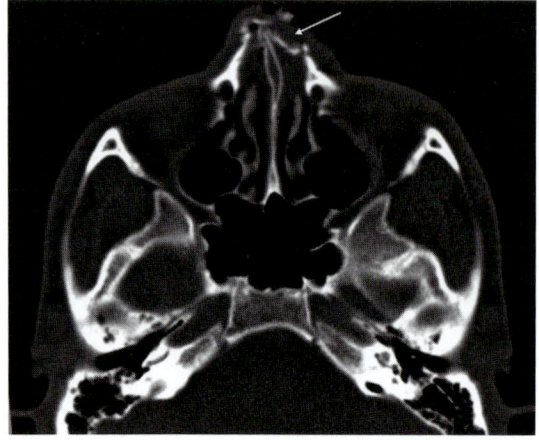

Fig. 1.33

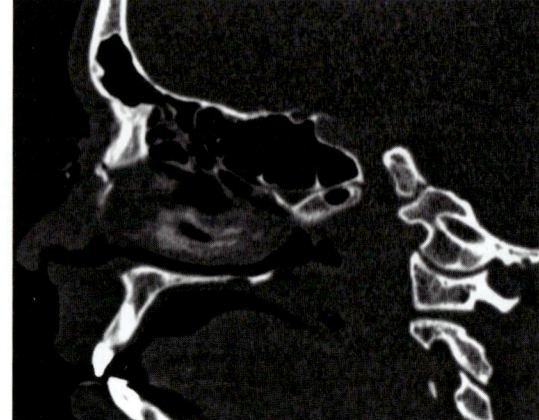

Fig. 1.34

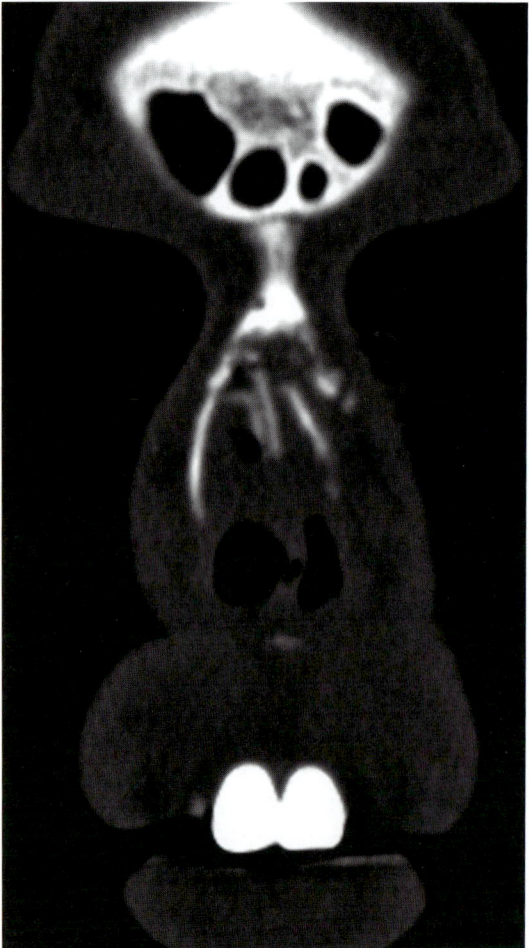

Fig. 1.35

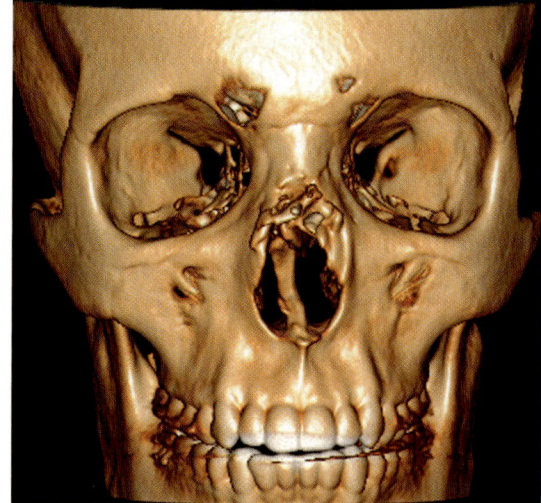

Fig. 1.36

An 11-year-old male presented with edema, ecchymosis, and nasal deformity after direct impact with a golf club.

Comment

Nasal fractures are defined as gaps in the nasal pyramid (nasal bones and cartilages + septum). Nasal are the most frequently fractured of all facial bones, particularly the septum cartilage, its union to the ethmoid's perpendicular plate and the nasal bones proper.

Nasal pyramid fractures are common in childhood and are usually derived from direct trauma such as house and sporting accidents (cycling), impact of hard objects on the face (in the sporting environment these would be hockey sticks, golf clubs, etc.), and road traffic accidents. It is important to distinguish simple nasal fractures from those occurring with fragment displacement or septum deviation since these may require surgical intervention.

Diagnosis is based on a good clinical history and examination. Quite frequently radiologic confirmation is not required for appropriate injury management.

Although plain radiographs (nasal bones lateral and occasionally Watters views) usefulness is debatable, it is carried out in unclear cases and for medicolegal reasons. Its value is even more limited in younger children with a larger proportion of non-ossified cartilage and where lack of cooperation may prevent an adequate study.

As some fractures may not be visible on plain radiographs, findings must be related to clinic history.

On the lateral view, the central beam should be directed through the film centered on the nasal bones, collimating it, thus the whole nose gets included. A good projection is one in which the nasal bones, including the anterior nasal spine, are represented in a strict lateral plane.

CT is more sensitive than conventional radiography in confirming fractures. It gives more information on situation, extension, damage to neighboring structures, and possible complications. However, as ionizing radiation should be avoided as much as practicable, CT is limited to selected cases such as complex facial trauma, suspicion of septal damage and, possibly, for appropriate surgical planning.

Radiology Findings

Due to the impact violence and clinical exam, a maxillofacial helicoidal CT was obtained in order to perform multiplanar reformatting and volumetric reconstruction.

The axial CT view (Fig. 1.33) shows a comminuted depressed fracture of the nasal bones and an associated septal fracture (arrow). A detached bony fragment is also seen.

Sagittal (Fig. 1.34) and coronal (Fig. 1.35) reformatted multiplanar views are useful to detail the fracture's trajectory, deviation, and angulation.

A 3D volumetric reconstruction (Fig. 1.36) can help in this case's surgical planning.

Case 1.10: Pool Drowning

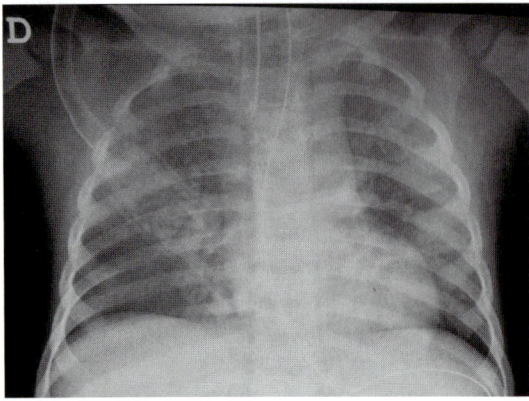

Fig. 1.37

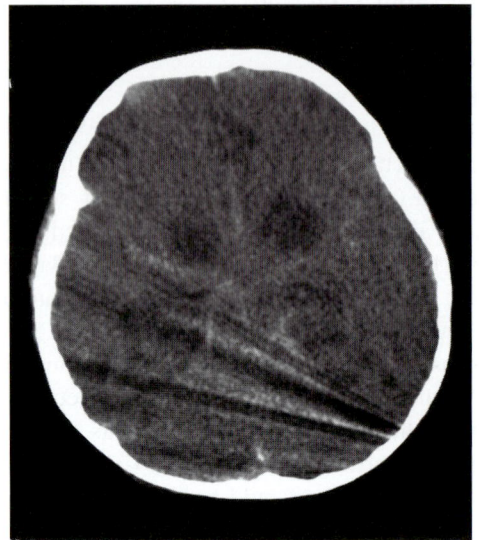

Fig. 1.38

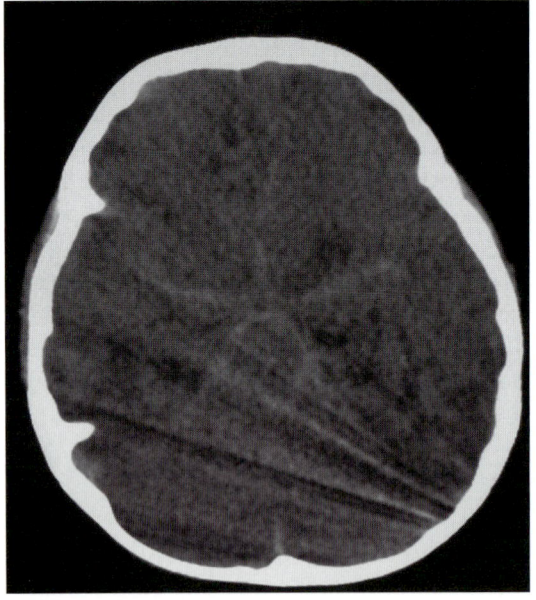

Fig. 1.39

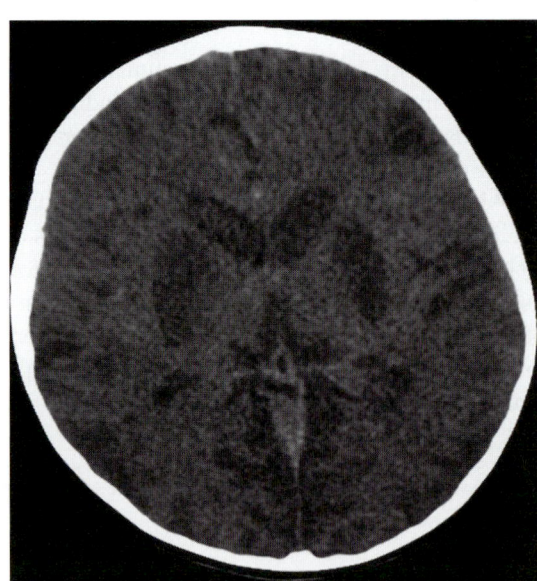

Fig. 1.40

A 5-year-old child was rescued from the bottom of a swimming pool. It was found in cardiac arrest. Advanced CPR cardiopulmonary resuscitation (orotracheal intubation included) was performed. Pulse regained after 26 min. Admitted to the Intensive Care Unit with a Glasgow Coma Scale of 3, midsized nonreactive pupils, without any spontaneous movement.

Comment

Drowning is the second most frequent cause of death in many countries. In cases where the subject survives, they are left with extremely severe neurological damage, so it truly represents a first-line public health problem.

The most frequent cause for pediatric (non-neonatal) hypoxic–ischemic injury is asphyxia, caused by either drowning or foreign body aspiration.

The term "*drowning*" is used if the patient dies in the 24 h following immersion, and "*near drowning*" if he/she survives that period of time. All these patients have suffered a relatively prolonged cerebral anoxia. The brain regions more severely affected are those with a high metabolic rate and high oxygen demand: basal ganglia, cerebellum, and cerebral cortex.

Typical findings in a hypoxic–ischemic cerebral CT are those of cerebral edema: sulci effacement and cistern definition loss in the brain's convexity, blurring of the white–gray matter interface due to cortex and basal ganglia hypodensity (which, in advanced cases, can turn into the "reversal sign" where, contrary to normal anatomy, the cortex is less dense than the white matter).

A "white cerebellum sign" is sometimes found where supratentorial hypodensity is in contrast with the more normally dense cerebellum.

The imaging technique that can demonstrate earliest hypoxic–ischemic lesion is MRI, with basal ganglia and cerebral cortex restriction on the diffusion sequence.

Prognosis depends on the cerebral anoxia time. Generally, patients arriving in hospital in coma have a negative outcome with severe neurological damage or death.

Radiological Findings

A conventional chest radiograph (Fig. 1.37) shows bilateral perihilar alveolar infiltrate consistent with pulmonary edema. It also confirms adequate endotracheal and nasogastric tube placement.

Transcranial Doppler alterations and anisocoria 10 h post cardiac arrest indicated to perform a CT study. It showed extensive cerebral edema, in both the posterior fossa with blurring of the cerebelar folia and 4th ventricle (Fig. 1.38), basal cisterns, hyperdense in comparison with adjacent parenchyma (pseudo-subarachnoid hemorrhage image) (Fig. 1.39), and blurring of supratentorial sulci (Fig. 1.40).

Bilateral basal ganglia and cortical hypodensity due to ischemia was also noted. Due to the evolving insult, the cortex is seen more hypodense than the white matter ("reversal sign").

Intracranial pressure continued to raise and the patient got worse. Brain death was established 18 h post admission.

Further Reading

Books

Harnsberger HC, Glastonbury CM, Michek MA, Koch BL (2010) Diagnostic imaging: head and neck, 2nd edn. Lippincott Williams&Wilkins, Philadelphia

Miloro M, Ghali GE, Larsen P, Waite P (2011) Peterson's principles of oral and maxillofacial surgery, 3rd edn. Pmph USA, Shelton

Osborn AG (2012) Osborn's brain: imaging, pathology, and anatomy. Amirsys. Lippincott Williams&Wilkins, Philadelphia

Robinson P (ed) (2010) Essential radiology for sports medicine. Springer, New York

Swartz JD, Loevner LA (2008) Imaging of the temporal bone, 4th edn. Thieme, New York

Websites

http://emedicine.medscape.com/article/872662-overview

http://pediatrics.aappublications.org/content/119/6/1242.full

http://radiopaedia.org/articles/hypoxic-ischemic-brain-damage

http://www.apcontinuada.com/es/traumatismo-craneoencefalico/articulo/80000152/

http://www.medigraphic.com/pdfs/orthotips/ot-2007/ot073e.pdf

Articles

Andronikou S, Van Toorn R (2009) The DWI 'reversal sign' of white matter hypoxic ischaemic injury in older children: an unusual MRI pattern for age. Pediatr Radiol 39(3):293–298

Brown CN, McKenna P (2009) A Wii-related clay-shoveler's fracture. Scientific World Journal 9:1190–1191. doi:10.1100/tsw.2009.134

Cakmakci H (2009) Essentials of trauma: head and spine. Pediatr Radiol 39(Suppl 3):391–405

Cusimano MD, Cho N, Amin K, Shirazi M, McFaull SR, Do MT, Wong MC, Russell K (2013) Mechanisms of team-sport-related brain injuries in children 5 to 19 years old: opportunities for prevention. PLoS One 8(3):e58868

Davison SP, Clifton MS, Davison MN, Hedrick M, Sotereanos G (2001) Pediatric mandibular fractures: a free hand technique. Arch Facial Plast Surg 3(3):185–189

Dubowitz DJ, Bluml S, Arcinue E, Dietrich RB (1998) MR of hypoxic encephalopathy in children after near drowning: correlation with quantitative proton MR spectroscopy and clinical outcome. AJNR Am J Neuroradiol 19(9):1617–1627

Egloff AM, Kadom N, Vezina G, Bulas D (2009) Pediatric cervical spine trauma imaging: a practical approach. Pediatr Radiol 39(5):447–456

Given CA 2nd, Burdette JH, Elster AD, Williams DW 3rd (2003) Pseudo-subarachnoid hemorrhage: a potential imaging pitfall associated with diffuse cerebral edema. AJNR Am J Neuroradiol 24(2):254–256

Han BK, Towbin RB, De Courten-Myers G, McLaurin RL, Ball WS Jr (1990) Reversal sign on CT: effect of anoxic/ischemic cerebral injury in children. Am J Roentgenol 154:361–368

Harris JB, Stern EJ, Steinberg KP (1995) Scuba diving accident with near drowning and decompression sickness. Am J Roentgenol 164(3):592

Holland AJ, Broome C, Steinberg A, Cass DT (2001) Facial fractures in children. Pediatr Emerg Care 17:157–160

Iida S, Matsuya T (2002) Paediatric maxillofacial fractures: their aetiological characters and fracture patterns. J Craniomaxillofac Surg 30(4):237–241

Junewick JJ (2010) Cervical spine injuries in pediatrics: are children small adults or not? Pediatr Radiol 40(4):493–498

Kaloostian PE, Kim JE, Calabresi PA, Bydon A, Witham T (2013) Clay-shoveler's fracture during indoor rock climbing. Orthopedics 36(3):e381–e383

Kang HM, Kim MG, Hong SM, Lee HY, Kim TH, Yeo SG (2013) Comparison of temporal bone fractures in children and adults. Acta Otolaryngol 133(5):469–474

Kim KA, Wang MY, Griffith PM, Summers S, Levy ML (2000) Analysis of pediatric head injury from falls. Neurosurg Focus 15:8(1)

Kjos BO, Brant-Zawadzki M, Young RG (1983) Early CT findings of global central nervous system hypoperfusion. Am J Roentgenol 141(6):1227–1232

Kubal WS (2012) Updated imaging of traumatic brain injury. Radiol Clin North Am 50(1):15–41

Logan M, O'Driscol K, Masterson J (1994) The utility of nasal bone radiographs in nasal trauma. Clin Radiol 49(3):192–194

Lustrin ES, Karakas SP, Ortiz AO, Cinnamon J, Castillo M, Vaheesan K, Brown JH, Diamond AS, Black K, Singh S (2003) Pediatric cervical spine: normal anatomy, variants, and trauma. Radiographics 23(3):539–560

Maxfield BA (2010) Sports-related injury of the pediatric spine. Radiol Clin North Am 48(6):1237–1248

Murthy NS (2012) Imaging of stress fractures of the spine. Radiol Clin North Am 50(4):799–821

Plaza Mayor G, Ferrando Alvarez-Cortinas J, de los Santos Granados G (2002) Pediatric temporal bone fractures. An Otorrinolaringol Ibero Am 29(3):237–246

Rao SK, Wasyliw C, Nunez DB Jr (2005) Spectrum of imaging findings in hyperextension injuries of the neck. Radiographics 25(5):1239–1254

Ulbrich EJ, Carrino JA, Sturzenegger M, Farshad M (2013) Imaging of acute cervical spine trauma: when to obtain which modality. Semin Musculoskelet Radiol 17(4):380–388

Muscle Strains and Avulsion Injuries

Rosa Mónica Rodrigo, Juan María Santisteban,
Javier Telletxea-Elorriaga, and Francisco Angulo

Contents

R.M. Rodrigo (✉)
Department of Radiology,
Resonancia Magnética Bilbao, Bilbao, Spain
e-mail: rmrodrigo@resonanciamagnetica.com

J.M. Santisteban
Medical Services, Athletic Club Bilbao, Bilbao, Spain

Department of Physiology, Faculty of Medicine
and Odontology, University of the Basque Country,
Bilbao, Spain

J. Telletxea-Elorriaga
Department of Bone Clinic, International SOS,
Bome Clinic, Bata, Equatorial Guinea

F. Angulo
Medical Services, Athletic Club Bilbao, Bilbao, Spain

R.M. Rodrigo et al., *Sports Injuries in Children and Adolescents*,
DOI 10.1007/978-3-642-54746-1_2, © Springer-Verlag Berlin Heidelberg 2014

Case 2.1: Anterior Superior Iliac Spine Avulsion Fracture

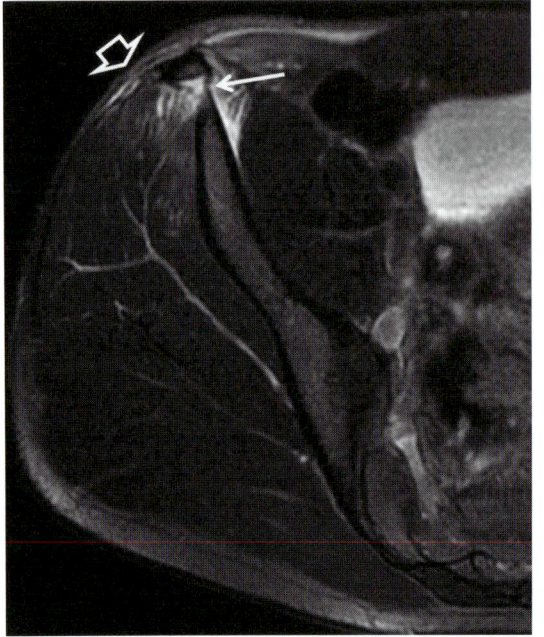

Fig. 2.1

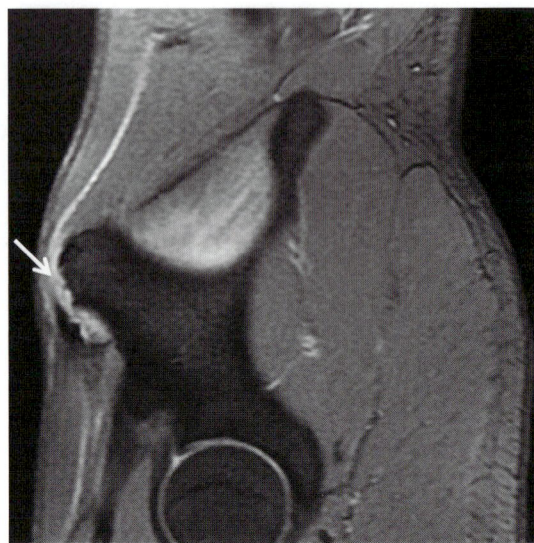

Fig. 2.2

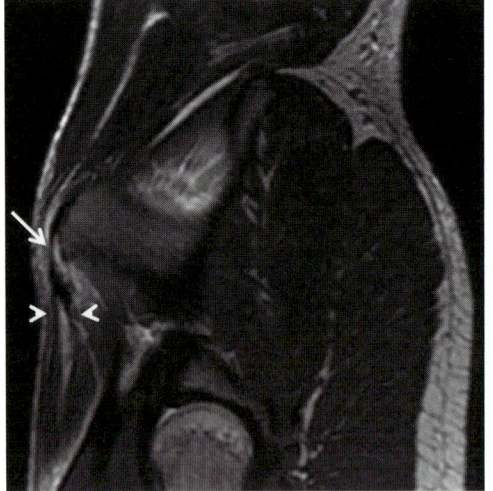

Fig. 2.3

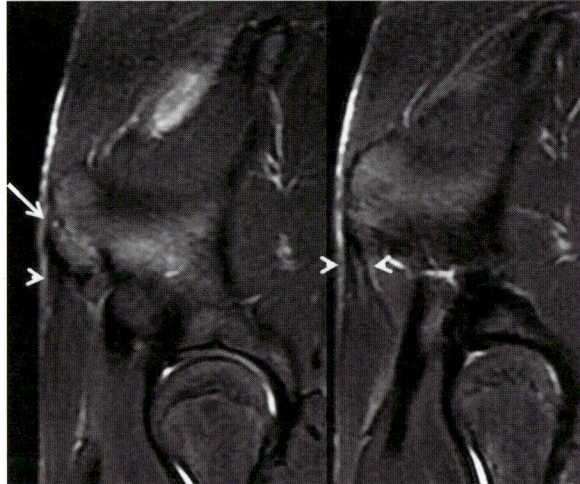

Fig. 2.4

A 17-year-old male soccer player complained of sudden pain and loss of function when running while training.

Comments

Avulsion fractures of the anterior superior iliac spine are rare injuries. However, they commonly affect the growing apophyses in adolescents undergoing vigorous activity.

In the immature skeleton, the apophysis (a cartilaginous growth center where a tendon attaches to bone) remains weaker than the attached musculotendinous unit until it fuses at the time of skeletal maturity and thus is more prone to fracture when the musculotendinous unit is suddenly and vigorously contracted.

The anterior superior iliac spine, which develops from an iliac crest's anterior apophysis, not normally fused until aged 20–25, is an insertion point for the sartorius muscle and part of the tensor fasciae latae. An avulsion fracture of the anterior superior iliac spine is most commonly due to forceful contraction or sudden repetitive actions of these muscles, as occurs when running or kicking a ball. Sprint athletes, soccer players, and gymnasts are the most frequently affected athletes due to the range of movements performed and sudden changes in direction required.

Plain radiographs are useful and the cheapest technique to diagnose this injury even though muscle insertions are not seen. MRI, CT, and sonography enable a more accurate diagnosis. MRI and sonography are a better choice than CT as they do not emit ionizing radiation.

The treatment of choice for this injury remains conservative: rest, analgesia, anti-inflammatories, and physical therapy; however, surgical treatment has been used depending on the degree of fracture displacement and the individual's rehabilitation requirements.

Patients frequently take long periods of time to recover. This particular soccer player took 61 days to return to competition.

Radiological Findings

Axial fat-suppressed T2-weighted FSE MR image (Fig. 2.1) shows the incomplete anterior superior iliac spine (ASIS) fracture, with the internal cortex still attached to the iliac crest (arrow). Subcutaneous edema (open arrow) and surrounding hematoma (slightly more hyperintense than muscle) are clearly appreciated. The gap at the fracture (arrow) is nicely seen in this sagittal fast gradient-recalled weighted MR image (Fig. 2.2).

Oblique fast T2-weighted MR image (Fig. 2.3) from the fracture's inner side clearly shows the integrity of the internal cortex (arrow). Sartorius and fascia latae tendon insertions (arrowheads) are seen attached to the avulsed apophysis.

The two continuous oblique fat-suppressed proton density-weighted MR images (Fig. 2.4) 4 months later show healing of the ASIS avulsion (arrow) with both tendon insertions (arrowheads) attached to it.

Case 2.2: Acute Avulsion Fracture of the Anterior Inferior Iliac Spine

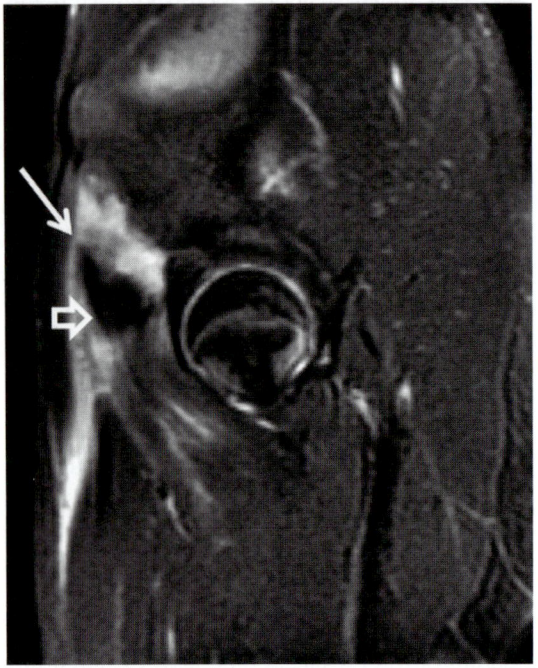

Fig. 2.5

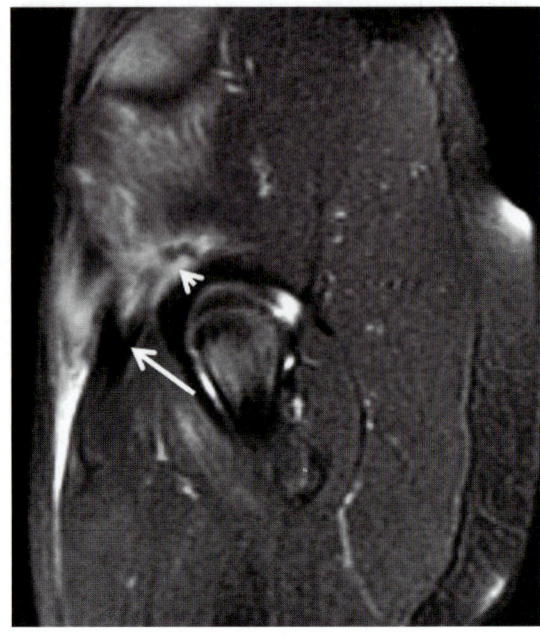

Fig. 2.6

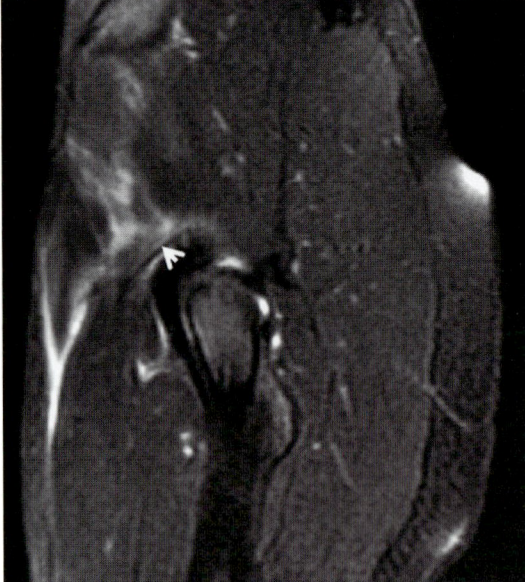

Fig. 2.7

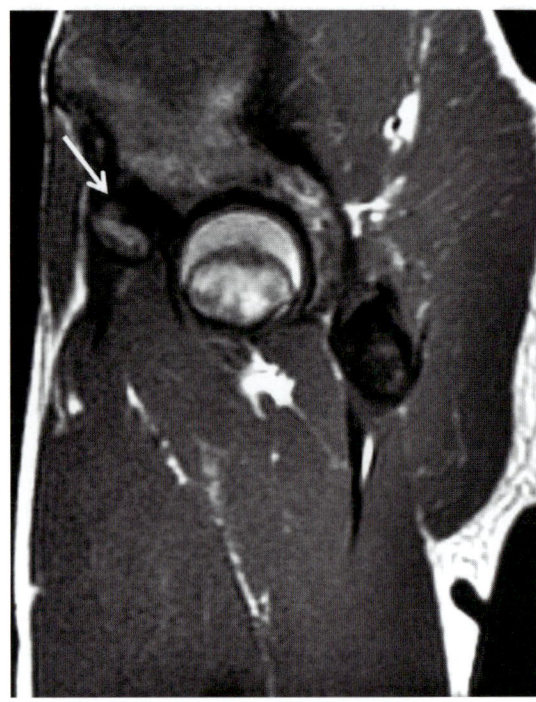

Fig. 2.8

A 15-year-old soccer player suffered a sudden groin pain when sprinting during preseason training on the beach. On examination, there was pain and loss of function on hip flexion.

Comments

Rectus femoris (RF) avulsion is not as common as its myotendinous junction injury which is commonly reported among adolescent athletes involved in kicking sports.

The anterior inferior iliac spine's apophysis (AIIS) begins to ossify between years 13 and 14 and it is not complete until years 16–18; therefore, this unfused apophysis in immature athletes is the weakest link in the muscle-tendon-bone chain.

The rectus femoris muscle has two proximal tendinous insertions above the hip: the direct (straight) head, arising from the anterior inferior iliac spine (AIIS), and the indirect (reflected) head, arising more inferiorly and posteriorly from the superior acetabular ring and hip joint capsule. Both heads form a conjoined tendon a few centimeters below their origins.

The apophysis' avulsion is an acute injury that typically occurs due to a single episode of violent eccentric contraction of the RF, as hip extends and knee is flexed (as happens in a case of an "empty kick"). Generally, displacement of the fragment is no more than 1.5 cm, and the lesion usually has a good outcome with conservative treatment alone but requires long periods of rest (this player took 83 days to return to competition). The indirect tendon can remain attached to its insertion during AIIS avulsion injury.

The typical crescent-shaped avulsed AIIS fragment is seen in plain radiograph, CT, sonography, and MRI, but the indirect tendon insertion is only seen on MRI, making it the technique of choice for this injury.

Imaging Findings

Fracture line with a mild displacement of the apophysis and direct tendon (open arrow) with edema and hemorrhage in surrounding tissues are seen in the first (Fig. 2.5) of these oblique sagittal fast T2-weighted MR images (parallel to the iliac wing). The hyperintense appearance of the apophysis cartilaginous compound (arrow) accounts for the loss of demarcation in this sequence.

Both the conjoined tendon (arrow) [showing integrity of myotendinous junction] and the partial disruption of the indirect tendon insertion (arrowhead) are seen in a contiguous external slice (Fig. 2.6). Fibers of this indirect tendon still attached to its insertion (arrow) are seen in the next contiguous external slice (Fig. 2.7).

In the sagittal proton density-weighted image (Fig. 2.8) taken 4 months later, the avulsed fragment is seen attached to the iliac crest with fibrous and ossified tissue. A retracted and mildly atrophic proximal rectus femoris muscle is also appreciated as the result of the injury.

Case 2.3: Anterior Inferior Iliac Spine Apophysitis Evolution

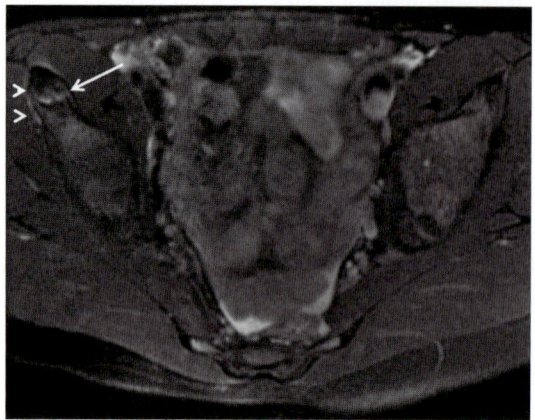

Fig. 2.9

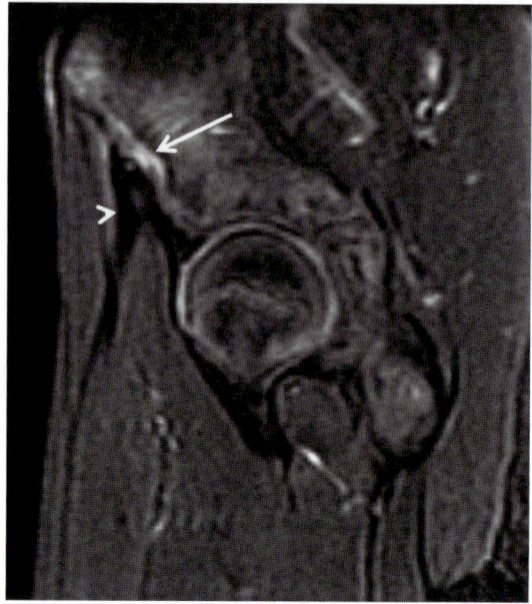

Fig. 2.10

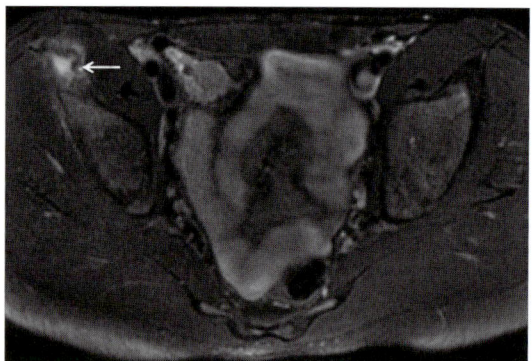

Fig. 2.11

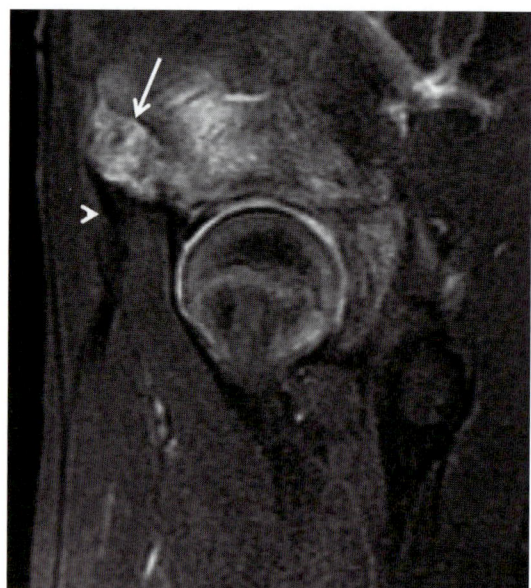

Fig. 2.12

A 13-year-old soccer player complained of groin pain when kicking right at the beginning of the season. After resting for 2 months, he gradually returned to play with no pain. A month later, he developed acute groin pain and loss of function during competition.

Comments

Anterior inferior iliac spine (AIIS) apophysitis is a chronic injury caused by repetitive microtrauma secondary to rectus femoris (RF) tendon traction from the apophyseal insertion. With more adolescents participating in highly competitive athletic activities, it has increased in prevalence over the past several decades.

The apophysis is a secondary ossification center that contributes to the size and shape of the bone, but not to its length. It is connected to the parent bone through an associated physis. Apophyses have also been termed "traction epiphyses." Distraction from chronic and repetitive musculotendinous pull is thought to stimulate chondrocyte proliferation or inflammatory cell hypertrophy at the physis, resulting in the apparent physeal widening and adjacent muscle edema seen on MRI, thus the term "apophysitis." The physis' hyaline cartilage adjacent to the apophysis is the site of less resistance until the apophysis is fused (age 16–18), so it is prone to be injured in adolescents overusing the rectus femoris muscle, such as soccer players and athletes.

Patients complain of vague pain over a period of time, not related to a specific episode of violent contraction. Aggravation of the apophysitis or avulsion of the anterior inferior iliac spine (AIIS) can occur with a sudden and vigorous contraction of the rectus femoris muscle, as was the case in this occasion.

Ultrasound is a better choice than plain radiography to detect this injury since it is capable of detecting non-ossification centers. Apophysitis is seen in MRI usually as a mild physeal widening of about 3–5 mm (as in this patient's initial episode) with hyperintensity on water-sensitive sequences, bone marrow edema, and, frequently, peripheral muscle edema.

The treatment usually consists of anti-inflammatory medication, activity modification, and rehabilitation. In this particular case, a complicated progress meant the patient required 9 months to return to practice.

Radiological Findings

The axial fat-suppressed T2-weighted image (Fig. 2.9) at the right AIIS shows a faint physeal widening (arrow) without displacement. Minimal edema (arrowheads) is seen surrounding the physis without bone marrow edema. The sagittal fat-suppressed T2-weighted image (Fig. 2.10) clearly shows the minimal widening of the physis and the direct rectus femoris tendon attached to the apophysis (arrowhead).

The same soccer player complained of pain 2 months later after vigorous contraction of the RF during competition. A wider apophyseal detachment (arrow) with marrow edema is clearly seen in the axial (Fig. 2.11) and sagittal (Fig. 2.12) fat-suppressed T2-weighted images. The tendon remains attached to the apophysis (arrowhead).

Case 2.4: Avulsion Injury of the Ischial Tuberosity

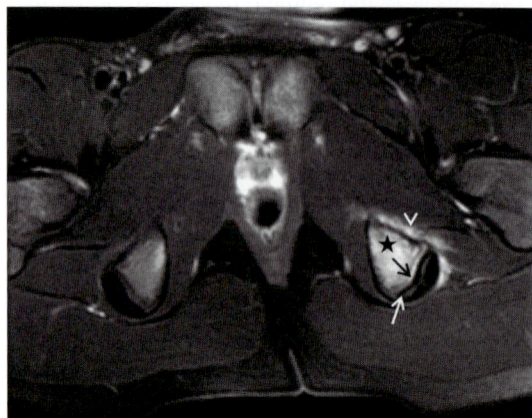

Fig. 2.13

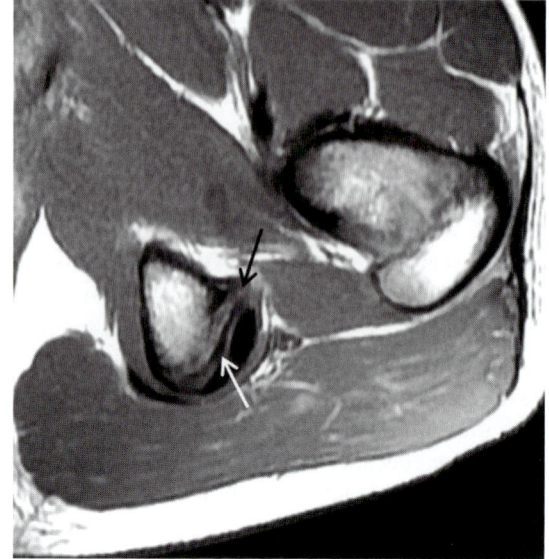

Fig. 2.14

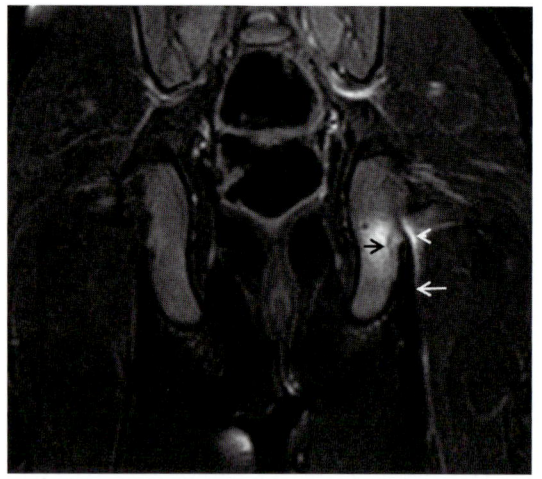

Fig. 2.15

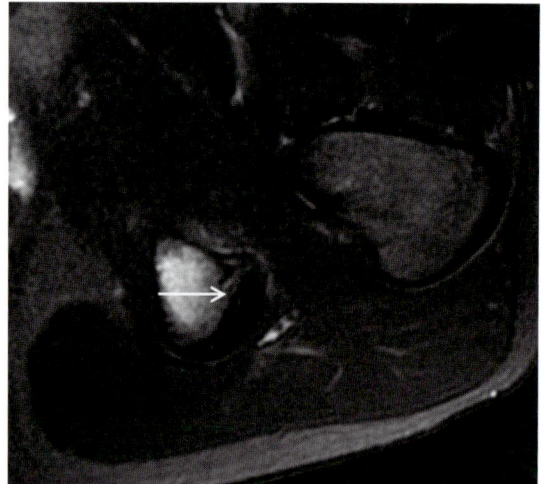

Fig. 2.16

A 14-year-old soccer player complained of sudden gluteal pain and difficulty in walking while competing.

Comments

Avulsion injuries of the ischial tuberosity are relatively common in adolescents and are commonly due to excessive eccentric contraction applied from the hamstring (HMS) muscles (long head of the biceps femoris, the semitendinosus, and the semimembranosus) that arise from it. These avulsions occur before the close of the ischial apophysis which is not completely fused until aged 20–25.

Patients usually complain of pain of sudden onset in the posterior gluteal or thigh region while the muscle is undergoing voluntary or involuntary eccentric contraction with the hip flexed and knee in extension. These injuries are common in soccer players, gymnasts, and dancers, among others.

With a mild (minor) apophyseal displacement, radiography sometimes does not provide conclusive information even though an elongated bony fragment (similar to the curve of the ischium) can occasionally be seen in oblique views (anteroposterior with 25–30° caudocranial beam inclination). MRI can be used to diagnose mild apophyseal displacement, but ultrasound can be more accurate for small cortical avulsions. If the displaced ossicle remains in close contact with the apophyseal cartilage, it can be completely reabsorbed inside the apophysis during the bone maturation process.

In larger lesions (avulsion greater than 2 cm), the apophyseal fragment tends to be displaced caudally, far away from the ischium, and can be transformed into a permanent ossicle with a spherical or oval shape with a thin cortical cover. Hypertrophied callus at ischium level and adjacent heterotopic bone should not be confused with major lesions.

Minor apophyseal displacements, as seen in this particular case, are treated with rest, icing, simple analgesics, protective weight bearing, and rehabilitation. This soccer player took 125 days to return to play. Surgical repair is indicated for either failed conservative treatment or for displacement greater than 2.5 cm.

Radiological Findings

The axial fat-suppressed T2-weighted image (Fig. 2.13) shows an elongated tiny bony fragment (white arrow) displaced from the left ischial tuberosity (asterisk) with extensive physeal (black arrow), ischial, and soft tissue edema (arrowhead). The avulsed fragment (white arrow) and periosteal stripping at the inner attachment (arrow) are clearly seen in a closer axial FSE proton density view (Fig. 2.14).

The coronal fat-suppressed T2-weighted image (Fig. 2.15) shows normal hamstring tendons (white arrow) with physeal (black arrow), ischial tuberosity, and soft tissue edema (arrowhead). Decreased bone marrow and soft tissue edema are seen in the axial fat-suppressed T2-weighted image (Fig. 2.16) taken 4 months later. The physis is undergoing fibrotic changes with no hyperintensity signal (arrow), while the avulsed fragment is not clearly defined.

Case 2.5: Avulsion Injury of the Tibial Tuberosity

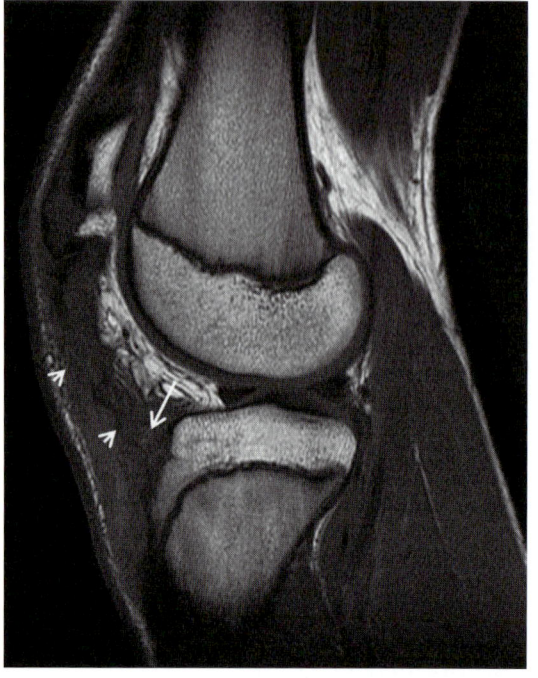

Fig. 2.17

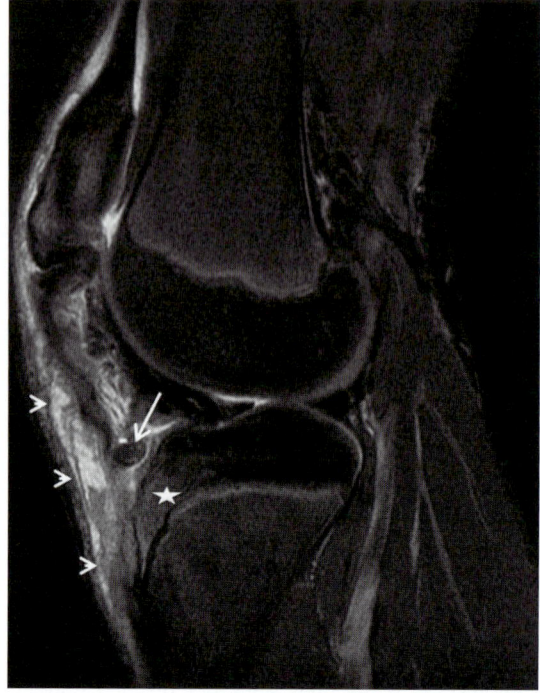

Fig. 2.18

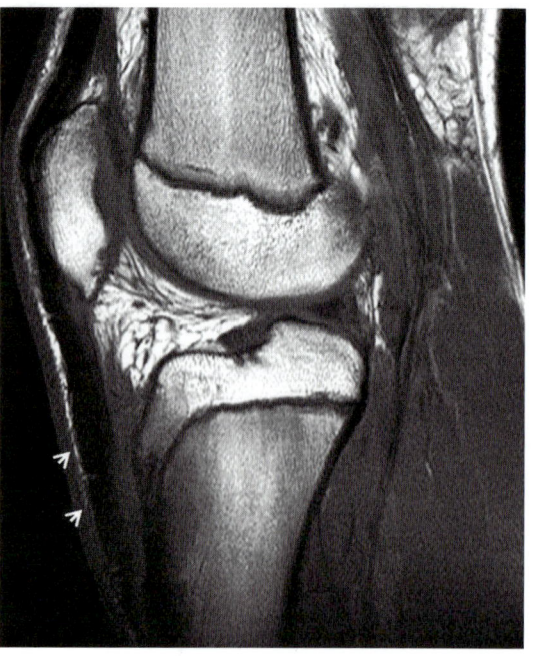

Fig. 2.19

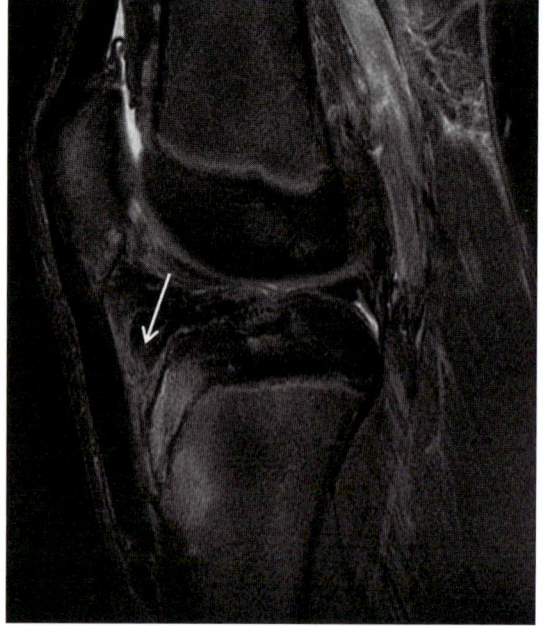

Fig. 2.20

A 17-year-old soccer player felt a pop below the knee after jumping to clear a ball and bouncing on the pitch. In previous weeks he had reported insidious pain over the anterior tibial tuberosity area secondary to probable Osgood-Schlatter disease.

Comments

Anterior tibial apophysis injuries in adolescents are uncommon. They are more frequent in males approaching skeletal maturity with well-developed quadriceps and in athletes with preexisting Osgood-Schlatter disease.

The tibial tuberosity develops from an ossification center appearing at ages 8–12 in girls and 9–14 years in boys. Fusion between the ossified tuberosity and tibial metaphysis is usually completed by ages 15 in girls and 17 in boys.

Avulsion fractures of the tibial tuberosity are classified by Watson-Jones into three types: *Type I*, the fracture line passes through the distal part of the tuberosity's physis lifting the ossification nucleus upwards; *Type II*, the fracture line is longer and involves the ossification nucleus and the proximal tibial physis, but does not enter the joint; and *Type III*, the fracture extends into the joint.

Types I and II are more common in younger athletes (12–14), type III occurs in older ones (15–17). This classification was modified by Ogden et al. to include displacement and comminution. Other types (IV and V) have been proposed.

These injuries are sustained during athletic activity involving jumping (basketball and high jump). Two possible mechanisms of injury are involved: violent knee flexion against a tightly contracting quadriceps (as in landing from a jump) or violent quadriceps contraction against a fixed foot (as in jumping). Patients complain of immediate pain and swelling with significant disability for standing and walking, as they cannot straighten the knee.

Plain radiographs in slight internal rotation (the tubercle is lateral to the midline) are sufficient for the diagnosis. MRI may be needed to detect associated knee injuries (patellar and quadriceps tendon, collateral ligaments, anterior cruciate ligament tears, etc.).

Closed management can be used in Types I and II with minimal displacement; open reduction and internal fixation is recommended for the rest.

This player underwent O.R.I.F (open reduction and internal fixation) with a good outcome, returning to competition 6 months later.

Radiological Findings

Sagittal T1-weighted (Fig. 2.17) and fat-suppressed T2-weighted images (Fig. 2.18) show a *Type I* injury with an ossification nucleus (large arrow) and an edematous patellar tendon (short arrows) avulsed and displaced proximally. Bone marrow (asterisk) and soft tissue edema (arrowheads) along the anterior knee plane are evident.

Sagittal T1-weighted (Fig. 2.19) and fat-suppressed T2-weighted images (Fig. 2.20) taken 6 months later after O.R.I.F. show the patellar tendon's integrity (small arrows) with retropatellar (large arrow) and bone marrow edema in the anterior tuberosity.

Case 2.6: Obturator Externus Injury

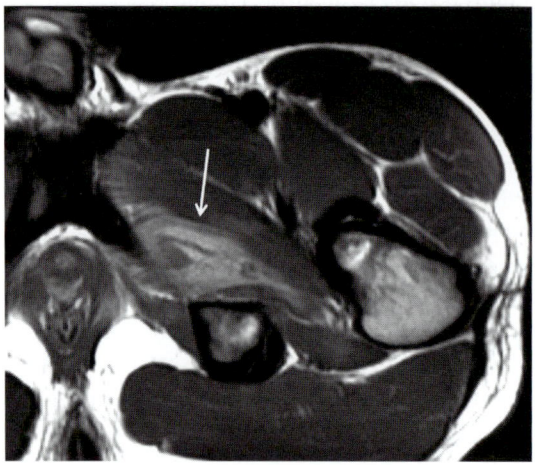

Fig. 2.21

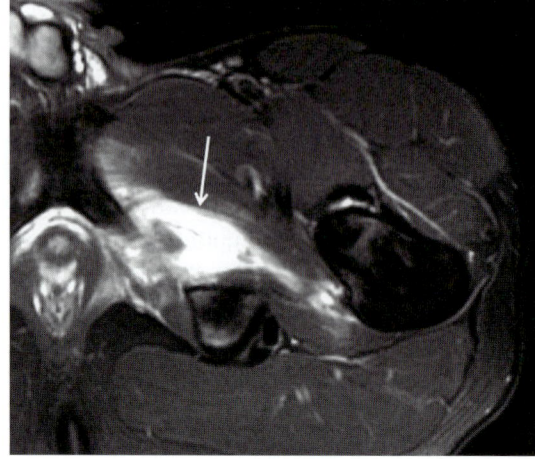

Fig. 2.22

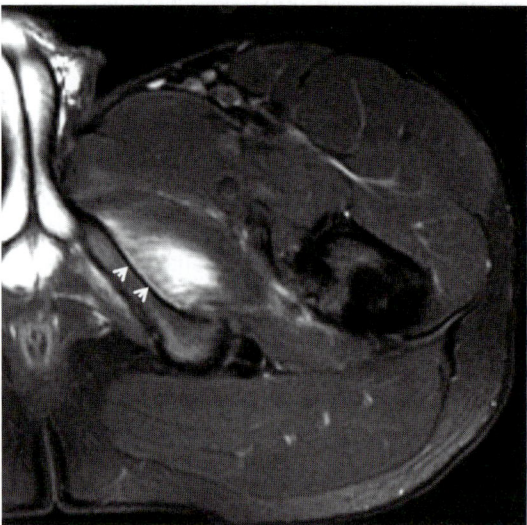

Fig. 2.23

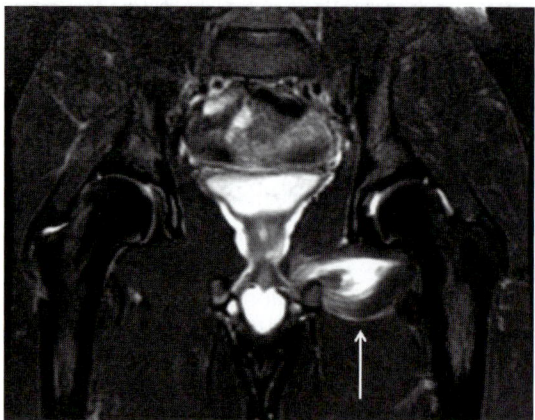

Fig. 2.24

A 17-year-old soccer player complained of acute groin pain (without ecchymosis or swelling) while training.

Comments

External hip rotator muscle strain injuries are rare in sports. They are most usually seen in soccer players. Although uncommon, they can incur into long recovery periods and can be misdiagnosed. They usually occur with the adduction and rotation of the hip, movements frequently practiced during soccer training. Initially, they are frequently misdiagnosed as adductor strain injuries, and although adductor stress tests provoke vague pain, it is the internal rotator hip test which elicits pain in the groin area (as the external hip rotator muscles are in tension). This does not occur in adductor strain injuries. A careful physical examination and MRI studies are needed if there is a suspicion of these lesions.

The external hip rotator muscles are: quadratus femoris, obturator (internus and externus), piriformis and gemellus (inferior and superior). In our experience, obturator (both internus and externus) injuries are the ones most frequently causing groin pain. The obturator externus arises from the external surface of the obturator membrane and its environment and, distally, ends in a tendon in the trochanteric fossa (on the posterior surface of the femur where the greater trochanter joins the neck). Obturator internus fibers arise from the inner surface of the obturator membrane and surrounding areas to reach the tip of the trochanteric fossa. Both muscles contribute to the lateral rotation and adduction of thigh at the hip. The internal obturator also participates in thigh abduction.

MRI provides an excellent tool for injury diagnosis of these muscles, which may be missed in ultrasound because of their deep location. Grade 1 injuries are seen as diffuse intramuscular edema. Grade 2 injuries are seen as intramuscular edema plus perifascial fluid beyond the muscle margin and hematoma. Grade 3 injuries are not common.

It took 16 days for this player to return to play.

Radiological Findings

The axial MR FSE proton density (Fig. 2.21) and FSE T2-weighted with fat suppression images (Fig. 2.22) show a Grade 2 injury with intramuscular hematoma along the obturator externus muscle fibers. A more caudal axial FSE T2-weighted with fat suppression image (Fig. 2.23) shows the extensive insertional fibers' edema (arrowheads) in the obturator membrane's external surface.

In the coronal MR FSE T2-weighted with fat suppression image (Fig. 2.24), the hematoma is clearly defined within the muscle belly. Some perifascial edema (arrow) is seen below the muscle.

Case 2.7: Rectus Femoris Indirect Tendon (Intramuscular or Central Aponeurosis) Strain Injury

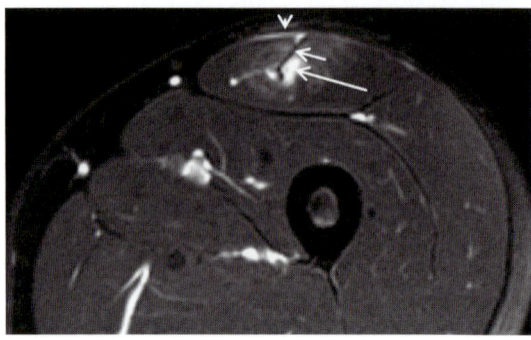

Fig. 2.25

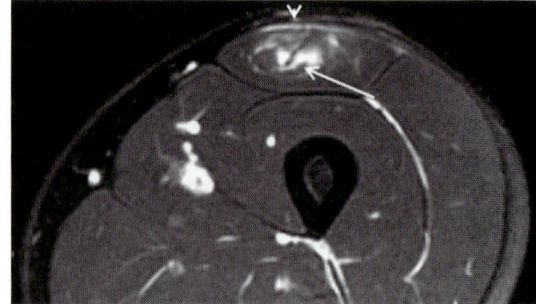

Fig. 2.26

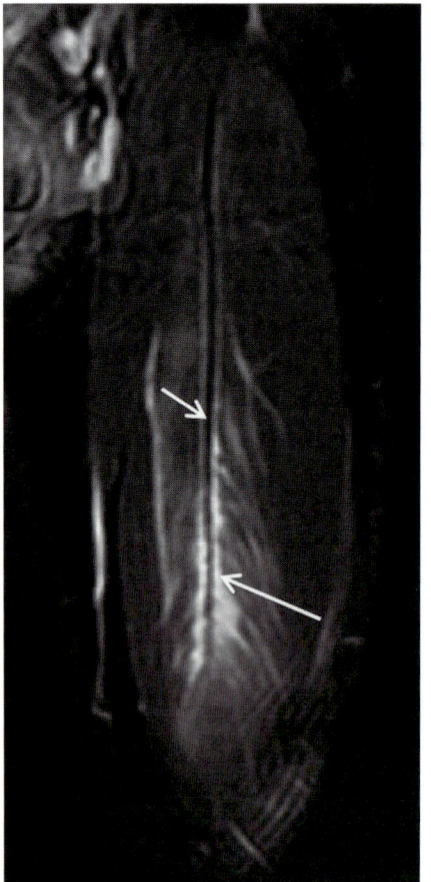

Fig. 2.27

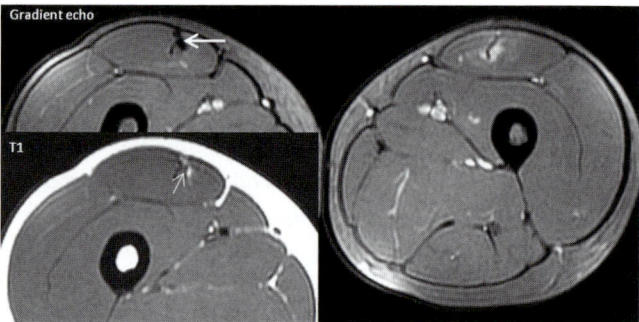

Fig. 2.28

A 17-year-old male soccer player complained of pain in the contralateral thigh (left) when trying to control the ball with his right leg during practice.

Comments

Rectus femoris (RF) injuries are common in soccer players. Unlike hamstring and tennis leg injuries, they are not related to age and can be seen in adolescent athletes. They are caused by an indirect mechanism during activities with eccentric contraction, such as sprinting and kicking.

The RF has a complex anatomy that defines the different injuries it sustains. It has two proximal tendinous insertions above the hip: the direct (straight) head, arising from the anterior inferior iliac spine (AIIS), and the indirect (reflected) head, arising more inferior and posteriorly from the superior acetabular ring and hip joint capsule. Both heads form a conjoined tendon a few centimeters below their origins. The *direct* head, forming most of the anterior part of the conjoined tendon, blends more distally with the RF's anterior fascia. The *indirect* head contributes to most of the posterior component of the conjoined tendon. It becomes a long intramuscular tendon (also called central tendon or central aponeurosis) just where the fibers of the inner RF belly insert. It extends approximately along two-thirds of the length of the muscle.

Indirect (reflected) tendon injuries are clinically classified as contractures as the pain is usually progressive and players generally complain of pain when kicking and sprinting.

Even though ultrasound is useful, MRI is excellent to accurately diagnose these injuries.

According to the traditional 3-grade system, they can be divided in three grades: *Grade I*, with feathery edema typically extending through the fibers inserting on both sides of the tendon while the tendon remains intact; *Grade II* (partial tears), architectural distortion of some of the muscle fibers with or without discontinuity of the intramuscular tendon (which is very interesting to point out); and *Grade III* (complete tears), complete disruption of the myotendinous junction, which in our experience is not seen. Variable hemorrhage/fluid amounts are usually seen surrounding the muscle below or (in more severe lesions) through the fascia and even between intermuscular planes.

These indirect injuries usually respond well to conservative therapy. Afterwards, a focal irregular scar of the indirect tendon is frequently seen at the rupture site.

It took 30 days for this particular player to recover.

Radiological Findings

Axial (Figs. 2.25 and 2.26 in a lower plane) and coronal (Fig. 2.27) fat-suppressed T2-weighted images show a Grade II injury with partial disruption (large arrow). Some of the muscle fibers inserting in the indirect tendon [which remains intact (short arrow)] are filled with fluid and hemorrhage and surrounded by edema. Anterior perifascial fluid is also seen (arrowheads).

Focal scar (thin arrow) and minimal fatty change (thick arrow) at the site of a prior injury to the right indirect RF tendon are seen in the axial T1-weighted and gradient echo images (Fig. 2.28) performed to study both thighs for comparison.

Case 2.8: Myofascial Rectus Femoris Lesion

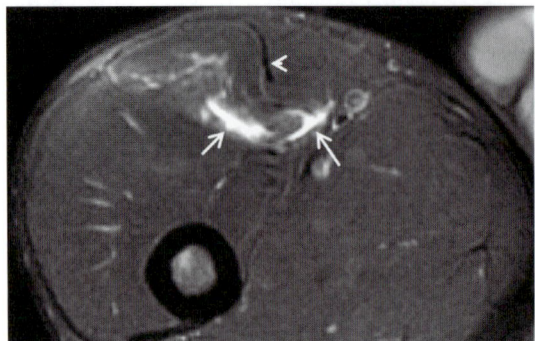

Fig. 2.29

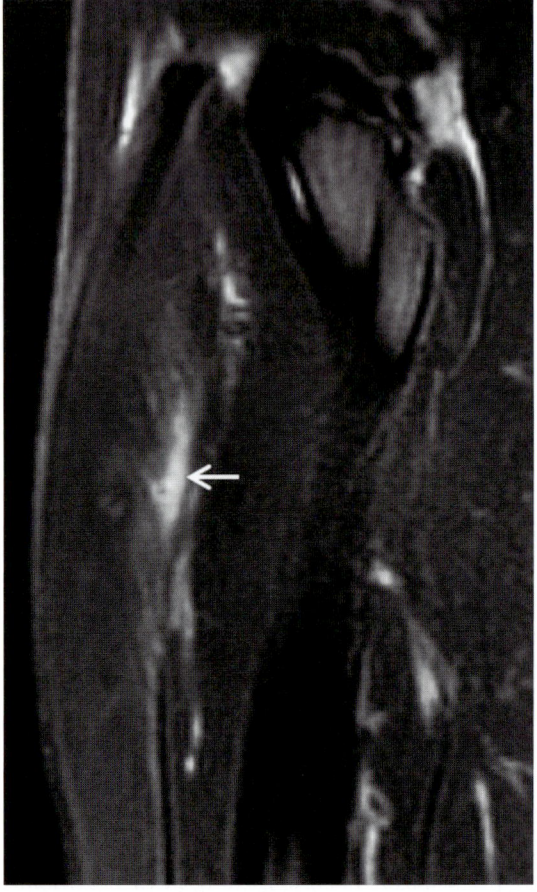

Fig. 2.30

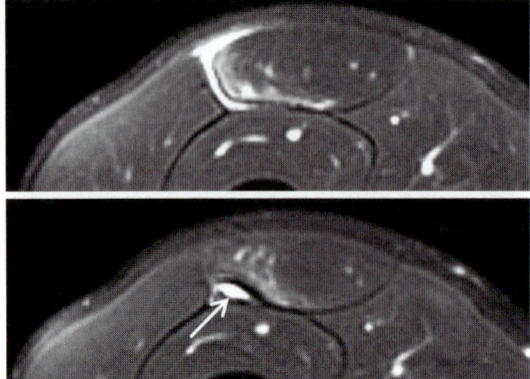

Fig. 2.31

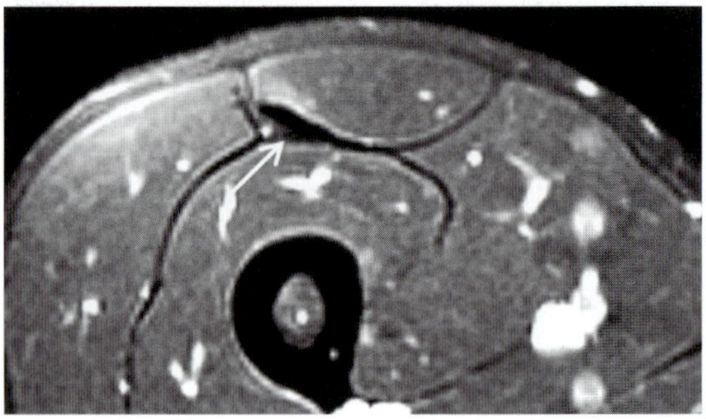

Fig. 2.32

A 17-year-old soccer player complained of mild thigh pain while sprinting.

Comments

Myofascial (MF) rectus femoris (RF) injury represents a different, less frequent entity than other RF myotendinous injuries. These are not centered along the myotendinous junction (MTJ); instead, they occur between the muscle fibers and the surrounding fascia which can sometimes be continuous with the MTJ.

Since unrelated to age, they are frequently seen in young soccer players. Athletes complain of mild insidious thigh pain when sprinting or kicking. The clinical examination elicits little pain on palpation, no swelling or muscle tension, and sometimes no pain against resistance. The pain worsens with the appearance of a seroma.

Although MF injuries can occur along any portion of the rectus femoris, they are more common in the proximal and middle two thirds. When these injuries happen anterior & very proximally, they may be difficult to differentiate from RF's direct head myotendinous injuries on MRI, and they may represent myotendinous injuries extending to the fascia. Myofascial injuries further down the rectus femoris are clearly differentiated from myotendinous injuries of the indirect head, as the edema and fluid are located eccentrically along the posterior and lateral aspect of the muscle and not centered along the indirect head's intramuscular tendon. Bilateral MF injuries can also be seen.

When the macroscopic fiber disruption is limited, the anterior and proximal MF injuries can be difficult to diagnose with ultrasound (the posterior and lateral injuries are easier to see). MR imaging shows edema and fluid within the muscular periphery with extension to the fascia. If the fascia is intact, the fluid may dissect along the fascia's undersurface creating an identifiable plane between muscle and fascia. If the fascia is disrupted, edema and fluid will extend beyond the muscle dissecting along the intermuscular planes. Deeper myofascial injuries, more common posterolaterally, have a greater tendency to reinjury and seroma formation if the player resumes training too soon after the original injury.

There are no studies specifying return to practice time with this type of injury, but in our experience, it takes fairly long to recover. This particular player took 33 days to return to competition.

Radiological Findings

Axial (Fig. 2.29) and sagittal (Fig. 2.30) fat-suppressed T2-weighted images show myofascial disruption along the posterior margin of the rectus femoris' middle third. Fluid is seen tracking along the fascia and the muscle belly (arrows). The RF's indirect MTJ remains intact (arrowhead).

These axial fat-suppressed T2-weighted images (Fig. 2.31) illustrate the evolution of a posterolateral MF injury in another player, showing seroma formation (arrow) 1 month later. The classical laminar hypointense scar (arrow) from this prior myofascial injury is nicely seen 3 months later (Fig. 2.32).

Case 2.9: Iliopsoas Strain Injury

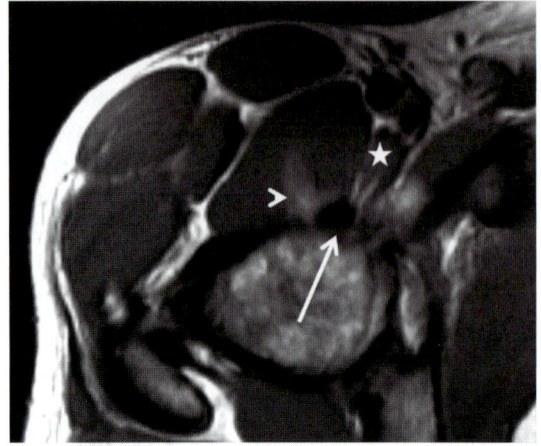

Fig. 2.33

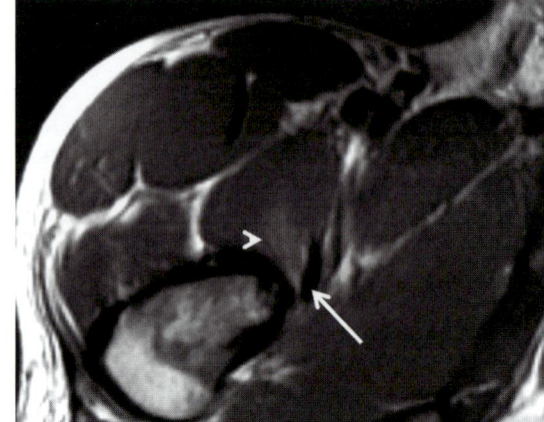

Fig. 2.34

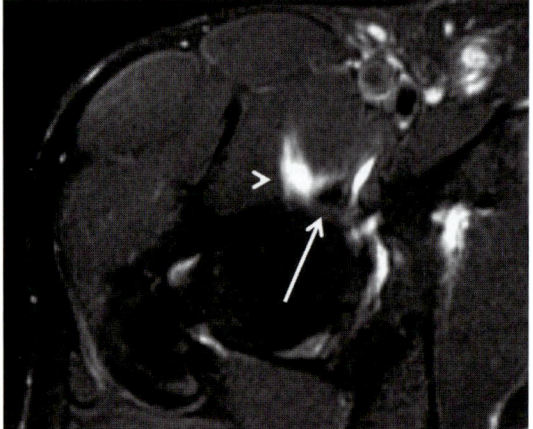

Fig. 2.35

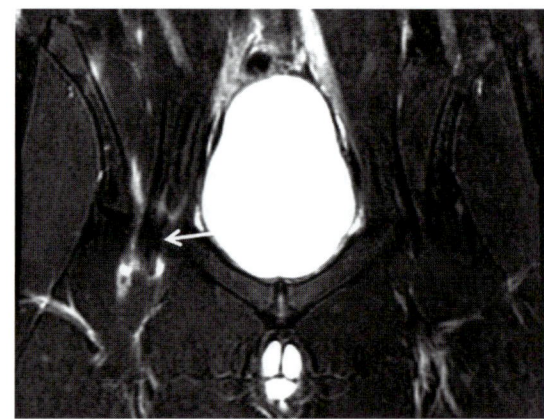

Fig. 2.36

A 17-year-old soccer player complained of acute groin pain after forced leg flexion while trying to control the ball during a game. He continued playing for a while but had to abandon the game afterwards.

Comments

Avulsion of the iliopsoas tendon with detachment of the lesser trochanter (prior to apophysis fusion) is the most common entity secondary to athletic injuries seen in children and adolescents. Nevertheless, iliopsoas *strain* injuries can also be seen although they are unusual. More severe tendon injuries (partial and completed tears) usually occur in older people.

The iliopsoas muscle strain injury can occur with forceful and sudden resistance to hip flexion (e.g., when a soccer player collides with another while kicking a ball). The main symptom is groin pain.

The *iliopsoas tendon* (*IPT*) *complex* includes the iliopsoas tendon itself (formed by crisscrossing fibers from the medial iliacus and psoas major tendon) attached to the lesser trochanter, the lateral portion of the iliacus muscle attached directly to the proximal femoral diaphysis (just distal to the level of the lesser trochanter) anterior portion, and, sometimes, a thin intramuscular tendon within the lateral iliacus separated from the ilio-psoas tendon by a fatty fascia cleft. The IPT unit acts as a thigh flexor and aids in lateral rotation of the hip.

Iliopsoas muscle strain injuries tend to occur at the MTJ (myotendinous junction). MRI is the technique of choice for diagnosis given this tendon's deep location within the hip. Without tendon rupture, edema is seen both intramuscularly and surrounding the iliopsoas tendon. The perilesional edema can even extend proximally between the iliacus bone and iliacus muscle. Radiologically, mild intramuscular edema can be confused with bursitis.

These strain injuries take long to recover. It took this particular player 45 days to return to full competition.

Radiological Findings

These two continuous axial proton density (Figs. 2.33 and 2.34) and FSE fat-saturated (Fig. 2.35) T2-weighted images demonstrate ill-defined edema at the iliopsoas myotendinous junction (arrow) with edema inside the lateral iliacus muscle (arrowhead). The psoas major is seen medially (asterisk).

The intact iliopsoas tendon with surrounding edema at the inguinal ligament level is appreciated in this coronal FSE fat-saturated (Fig. 2.36) T2-weighted image.

Case 2.10: Snapping Iliopsoas Tendon (Internal Snapping Hip)

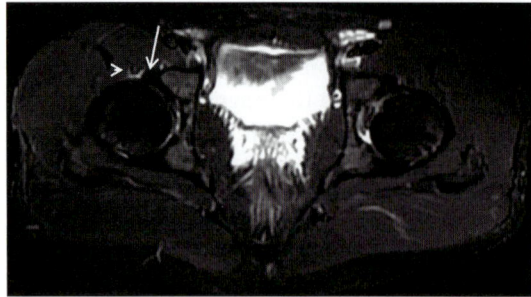

Fig. 2.37

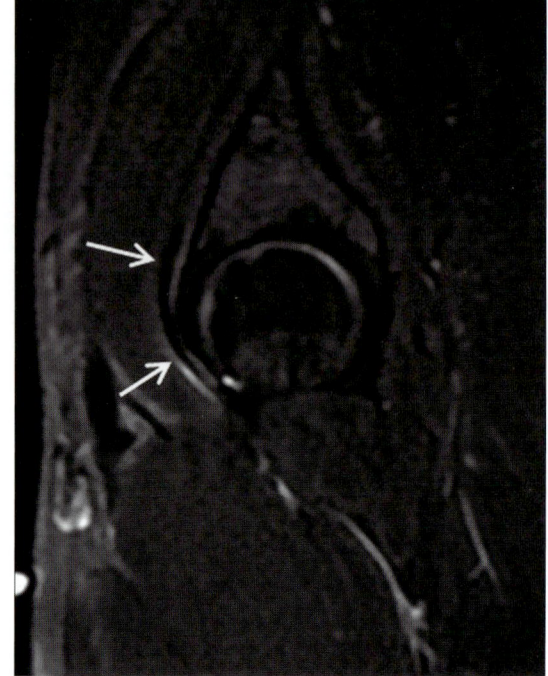

Fig. 2.38

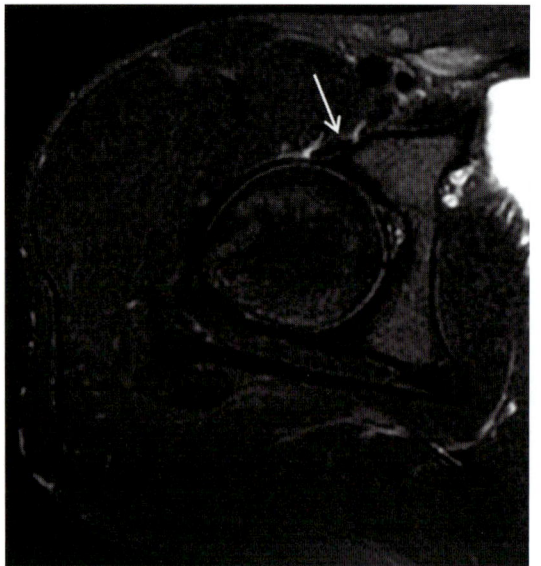

Fig. 2.39

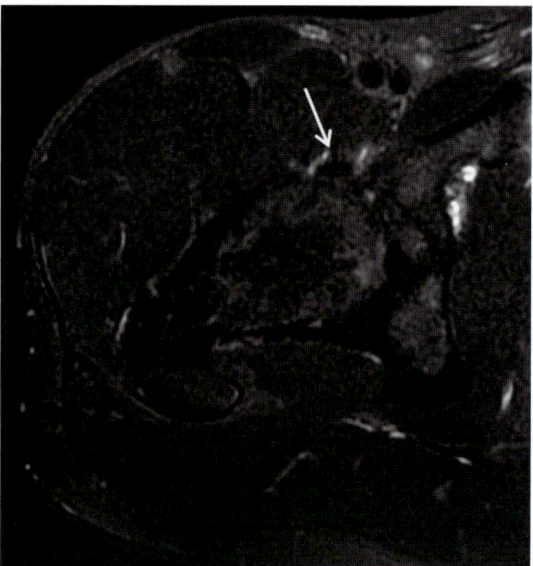

Fig. 2.40

A 17-year-old soccer player complained of deep anterior right groin pain while training. He felt internal snapping with different hip motions.

Comments

Snapping hip syndrome is a common cause of pain in young athletes performing a wide range of hip movements that usually demand repeated elevation of the leg over the horizontal line in adduction, as in karate and ballet.

Causes of snapping hip may be intra-articular (e.g., labral tears, chondral defect, loose bodies) and extra-articular (related to the iliopsoas tendon or iliofemoral ligament anteriorly and iliotibial band or gluteus maximus laterally). The extra-articular syndrome has also been divided in external (caused by iliotibial band or gluteus maximus) and internal (caused by the iliopsoas tendon). The iliopsoas tendon is suggested as the most common cause of snapping hip. There are three proposed mechanisms to explain this: catching between the tendon and its muscle, contact between the tendon and the iliopectineal eminence, or contact with the lesser trochanter ("friction syndrome").

Patients complain of pain and usually an audible or perceptible snap during specific hip movements, most frequently when the hip moves from flexion-abduction-external rotation (frog-leg position) to neutral. Some athletes may even experience a painless internal snapping syndrome with audible snap.

Sonography has emerged as the technique of choice to examine the iliopsoas tendon because it allows both static and dynamic evaluation of soft tissues around the hip joint. However, some athletes may complain of mild pain without an audible snap, and MR can be useful in ruling out intra-articular pathology and confirming the diagnosis. MRI tends to show a mild edema around the iliopsoas tendon without other signs of tendinopathy.

An accurate diagnosis is essential to decide on the appropriate treatment. It usually includes physical therapy with rest and analgesics. A combination of corticosteroid injection and local anesthetic into the iliopsoas bursa may be beneficial to relieve symptoms. Other treatments are rarely necessary.

Athletes normally return to activity after short periods of time. This particular soccer player was able to return to competition in 7 days, although he still required physical therapy.

Radiological Findings

A STIR-weighted image (Fig. 2.37) shows mild edema (arrowhead) surrounding the right iliopsoas tendon (arrow) in comparison with the left one. The sagittal FSE fat-suppression (Fig. 2.38) T2-weighted image shows the normal right iliopsoas tendon (arrows) with surrounding edema at the hip joint level.

The two continuous FSE fat-suppression T2-weighted images (Figs. 2.39 and 2.40) with smaller field of view nicely show the mild edema surrounding the right iliopsoas tendon (arrow) anterior to the hip joint.

Further Reading

Books

Balius R, Pedret C (2013) Lesiones musculares en el deporte. Panamerica, Madrid

Campbell WC, Canale ST, Beaty JH (2008) Campbell's operative orthopaedics, 11th edn. Mosby/Elsevier, Philadelphia

Karantas AH (2011) Sports injuries in children and adolescents. Springer, Berlin/Heidelberg

Martino F, Defilippi C, Caudana R (2009) Imaging of pediatric bone and joint trauma. Springer-Verlag, Italia

Lopes S, Machado M, Beber B (2013) Joint imaging in childhood and adolescence. Springer-Verlag, Berlin/Heidelberg

Websites

http://www.radiologyeducation.com
www.rad.washington.edu/academics/academic-sections/msk
www.radiolopolis.com
www.radsource.us
www.wheelessonline.com

Articles

Balius R, Maestro A, Pedret C, Estruch A, Mota J, Rodriguez L, García P, Mauri E (2009) Central aponeurosis tears of the rectus femoris: practical sonographic prognosis. Br J Sports Med 43:818–824. doi:10.1136/bjsm.2008.052332

Bianchi S, Martinoli C, Waser NP, Bianchi-Zamorani MP, Federici E, Fasel J (2002) Central aponeurosis tears of the rectus femoris: sonographic findings. Skeletal Radiol 31:581–586

Blankenbaker DG, De Smet AA (2010) Hip injuries in athletes. Radiol Clin North Am 48:1155–1178

Bui KL, Iaslan H, Recht M, Sundaram M (2008) Iliopsoas injury: an MRI study of patterns and prevalence correlated with clinical findings. Skeletal Radiol 37:245–249

Deslandes M, Guillin R, Cardinal E, Hobden R, Bureau NJ (2008) The snapping iliopsoas tendon: new mechanisms using dynamic sonography. AJR Am J Roentgenol 190:576–581

Dhinsa BS, Jalgaonkar A, Mann B, Butt S, Pollock R (2011) Avulsion fracture of the anterior superior iliac spine: misdiagnosis of a bone tumour. J Orthopaed Traumatol 12:173–176

Frey S, Hosalkar H, Cameron DB, Heath A, Horn BD, Ganley TJ (2008) Tibial tuberosity fractures in adolescents. J Child Orthop 2:469–474

Gamradt SC, Brophy RH, Barnes R, Warren RF, Byrd JWT, Kelly BT (2009) Nonoperative treatment for proximal avulsion of the rectus femoris in professional American football. Am J Sports Med 37(7):1370–1374

Gyftopoulos S, Rosenberg ZS, Schweitzer ME, Bordalo-Rodriguez M et al (2008) Normal anatomy and strains in deep musculotendinous junction of the proximal rectus femoris: MRI features. AJR Am J Roentgenol 190:w182–w186 (web exclusive article)

Hasselman CT, Best TM, Hughes C, Martinez S, Garret W (1995) An explanation for various rectus femoris strain injuries using previously undescribed muscle architecture. Am J Sports Med 23:493–499

Hébert KJ, Laor T, Divine JG, Emery KH, Wall EJ (2008) MRI appearance of chronic stress injury of the iliac crest apophysis in adolescent athletes. AJR Am J Roentgenol 190:1487–1491

Hsu JM, Fischer DA, Wright RW (2005) Proximal rectus femoris avulsions in national football league kickers. A report of 2 cases. Am J Sports Med 33(7):1085–1087

Kassarjian A, Rodrigo RM, Santisteban JM (2012) Current concepts in MRI of rectus femoris musculotendinous (myotendinous) and myofascial injuries in elite athletes. Eur J Radiol 81:3763–3771

Kaymaz B, Eroğlu M (2012) Avulsion fracture of the anterior inferior iliac spine in an uncommon way: a rare case. J Clin Exp Invest 3(2):267–269

Kerssemakers SP, Fotiadou AN, De Jonge MC, Karantanas AH, Maas M (2009) Sport injuries in the paediatric and adolescent patient: a growing problem. Pediatr Radiol 39:471–484

Kocher MS, Tucker R (2006) Pediatric athlete hip disorders. Clin Sports Med 25:241–253

Le Gall F, Carling C, Reilly T (2007) Biological maturity and injury in elite youth football. Scand J Med Sci Sports 17:564–572

Lecouvet FE, Demondion X, Leemrijse T, Vande Berg BC, Devogelaer JP, Malghem J (2005) Spontaneous rupture of the distal iliopsoas tendon: clinical and imaging findings, with anatomic correlations. Eur Radiol 15:2341–2346

McKoy BE, Stanitski CL (2003) Acute tibial tubercle avulsion fractures. Orthop Clin North Am 34:397–403

Mendiguchia J, Alentorn-Geli E, Idoate F, Myer GD (2013) Rectus femoris muscle injuries in football: a clinically relevant review of mechanisms of injury, risk factors and preventive strategies. Br J Sports Med 47(6):359–366. doi:10.1136/bjsports-2012-091250

Ouellette H, Thomas BJ, Nelson E, Torriani M (2006) MR imaging of rectus femoris origin injuries. Skeletal Radiol 35:665–672

Pesl T, Havranek P (2008) Acute tibial tubercle avulsion fractures in children: selective use of the closed reduction and internal fixation method. J Child Orthop 2:353–356

Polster JM, Elgabaly M, Lee H, Klika A, Drake R, Barsoum W (2008) MRI and gross anatomy of the iliopsoas tendon complex. Skeletal Radiol 37:55–58

Vandervliet EJ, Vanhoenacker FM, Snoeckx A et al (2007) Sports-related acute and chronic avulsion injuries in children and adolescents with special emphasis on tennis. Br J Sports Med 41:827–831

Yee PK, Poon KC, Chiu SY (2012) Simultaneous bilateral patellar tendon avulsion in an adolescent. Hong Kong Med J 18:530–532

Bone Fractures

3

José Martel, Silvia Martín, Ernesto Rivera,
and Ángel Bueno

Contents

J. Martel (✉) • Á. Bueno
Department of Radiology,
Hospital Universitario Fundación Alcorcón,
Madrid, Spain
e-mail: jmartel@fhalcorcon.es

S. Martín
Department of Radiology,
Hospital Son Llàtzer, Palma de Mallorca, Spain

E. Rivera
Department of Radiology,
Hospital Quirón, Málaga, Spain

R.M. Rodrigo et al., *Sports Injuries in Children and Adolescents*,
DOI 10.1007/978-3-642-54746-1_3, © Springer-Verlag Berlin Heidelberg 2014

Case 3.1: Scaphoid Nonunion

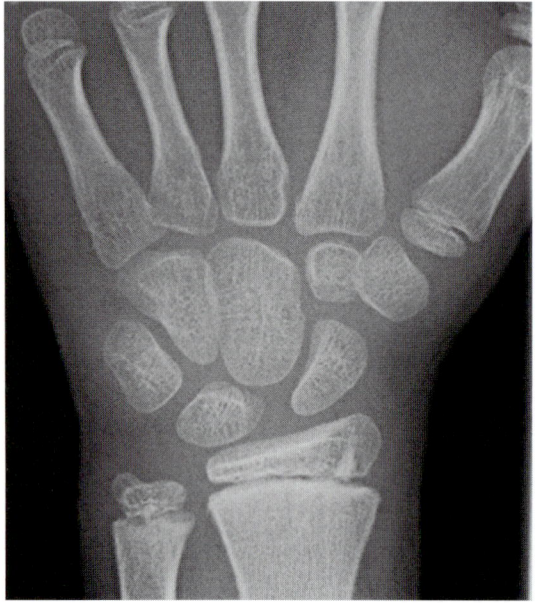

Fig. 3.1

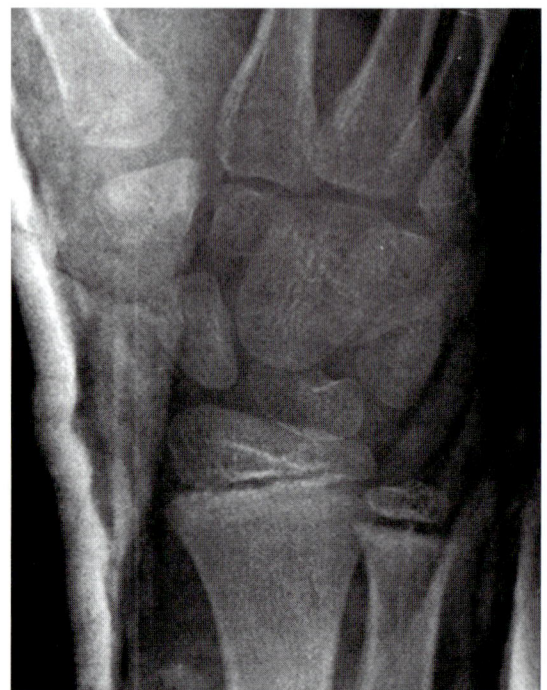

Fig. 3.2

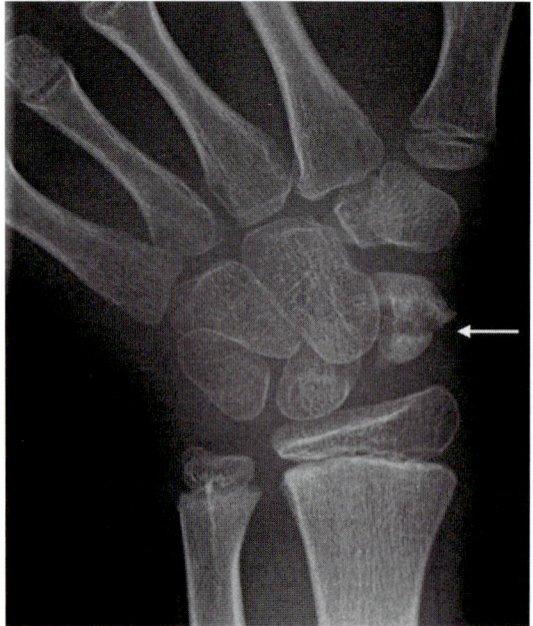

Fig. 3.3

Fig. 3.4

An 11-year-old male roller hockey player fell onto his outstretched hand and complained of wrist pain.

Comments

Scaphoid fractures are rare in children and adolescents. The large amount of cartilage present in the scaphoid during development makes it less susceptible to fractures. Their incidence has increased, probably due to sports and leisure activity changes in the younger population.

Nonunion of pediatric scaphoid fractures are extremely uncommon. Although investigators have attributed this complication to missed or wrong diagnosis, nonunion may develop even in appropriately managed scaphoid fractures.

Clinical signs are swelling, painfully limited wrist motion, tenderness over the anatomical snuffbox, and pain with axial loading of the first ray.

Plain films are the initial radiological study of choice: posteroanterior, lateral, oblique, and posteroanterior with ulnar deviation views should be obtained.

If a scaphoid fracture is undetected on the initial radiographs, treatment should include immobilization in a short-arm thumb cast, followed by radiological reassessment after 2 weeks. MRI and CT could be useful in selected patients.

There is no agreement about the standard treatment method. Extended conservative treatment may be an alternative in the youngest adolescents, but most authors recommend internal fixation with iliac crest bone grafting.

Imaging Findings

The initial plain film was normal (Fig. 3.1). After a 2-week cast immobilization, a new radiograph was obtained and was also reported as normal (Fig. 3.2). Despite the patient being asymptomatic, his treating physician ordered a new radiograph after two further weeks. For unknown reasons, he did not return for follow-up until 6 months later. Radiograph (Fig. 3.3) showed nonunion of the scaphoid's waist (arrow).

Coronal fat-suppressed T1-weighted image after intravenous gadolinium administration (Fig. 3.4) showed normal contrast enhancement in both fragments. Screw fixation with iliac crest bone grafting was performed with very good results.

Case 3.2: Early Closure of the Distal Tibial Physis Secondary to Epiphysiolysis Grade I

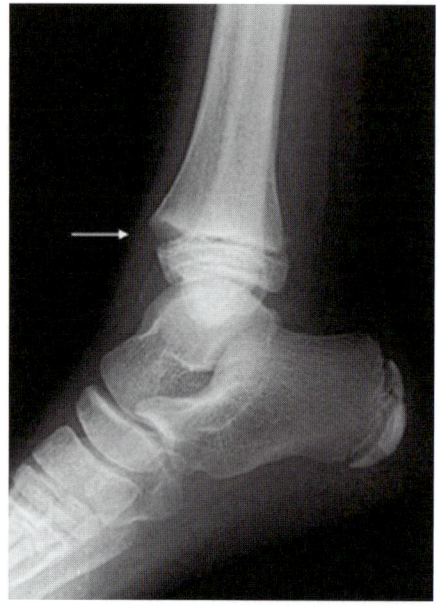

Fig. 3.5

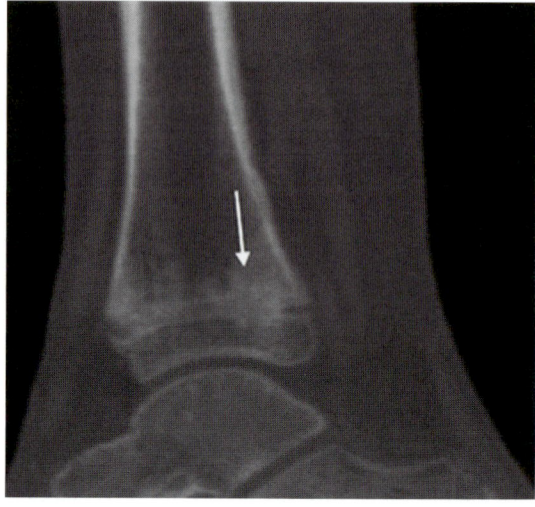

Fig. 3.6

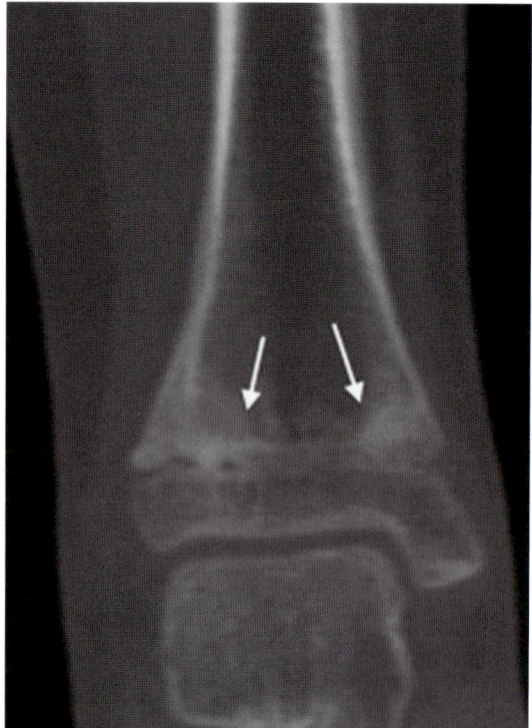

Fig. 3.7

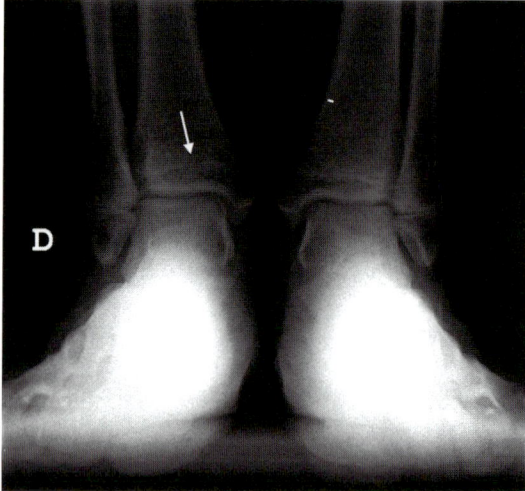

Fig. 3.8

An 11-year-old football player suffered a right ankle sprain pain. The clinical examination showed pain, swelling, and a slight deformity. Sensitivity and pulses were preserved.

Comments

Epiphysiodesis (premature epiphysis/diaphysis union, resulting in growth cessation) is a rare complication of epiphysiolysis. Usually seen in Salter-Harris type IV and exceptionally in type I fractures (as in our case).

Epiphysiodesis can be central, peripheral, or longitudinal. It requires surgical intervention when the physeal bridge gives cause to a shortening greater than 2 cm affecting less than 50 % the size of the physis.

Imaging Findings

A right ankle radiograph (Fig. 3.5) showed a type I epiphysiolysis (arrows).

It was treated with a splint for 6 weeks. After removal, the patient presented good mobility with a slight ankle edema but no other symptoms.

Two weeks later, the patient returned, limping with pain and showing mild edema in his ankle.

A CT (Figs. 3.6 and 3.7) of the right ankle showed a concentric periosteal reaction at the distal tibial metaphysis, accompanied by sclerosis and bony bridge formation in the physis center (arrows).

As the patient was asymptomatic when the CT was performed, the treatment was conservative.

Two years later, a plain radiograph (Fig. 3.8) showed early closure of the right tibial metaphysis (as compared with the contralateral side) and 1 cm of dysmetria of the lower extremities. The patient was asymptomatic.

Case 3.3: Proximal Femur Epiphysiolysis

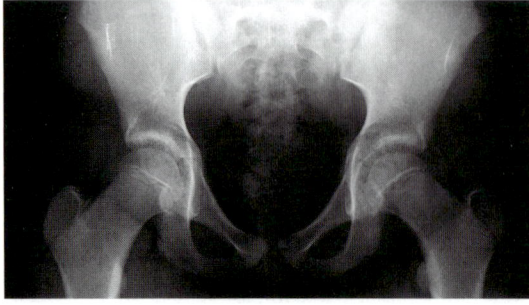

Fig. 3.9

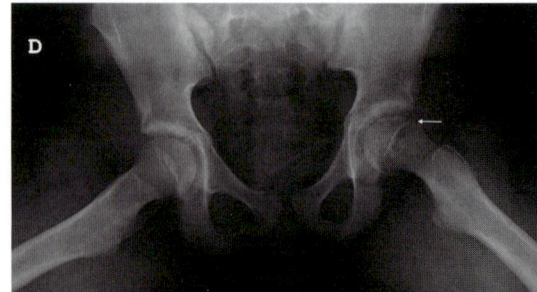

Fig. 3.10

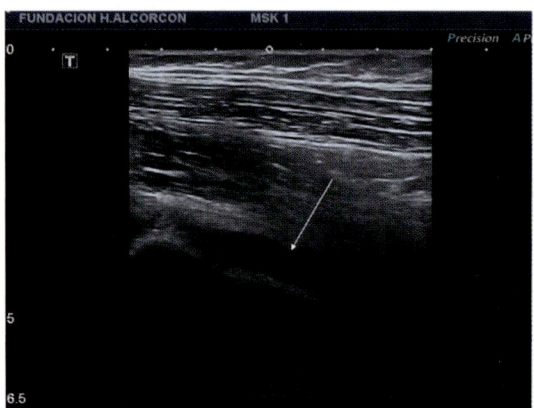

Fig. 3.11

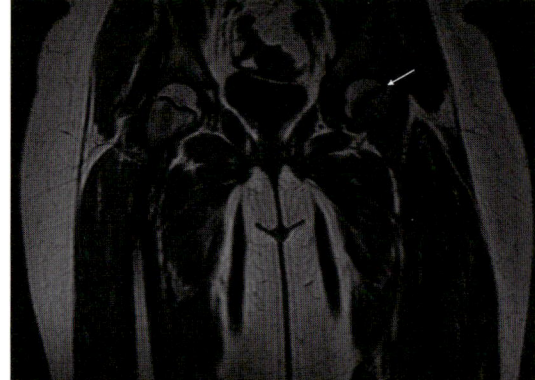

Fig. 3.12

A 10-year-old female practicing rhythmic gymnastics presented with a history of limping for 1 month, which had worsened in the previous week and was accompanied by significant functional impairment. There was no clear history of trauma.

Comments

Epiphysiolysis, or slipped upper femoral epiphysis, is rare and is the result of chronic repetitive trauma to the proximal femoral growth plate.

The radiographic changes may be subtle. Frog-leg lateral views of the hip demonstrate displacement better than standard anteroposterior views.

Malalignment of the femoral neck and epiphysis could be difficult to detect in ultrasound although effusion fluid can be seen around the metaphysis.

Magnetic resonance imaging depicts the typical features with widening of the growth plate associated with high signal on STIR sequences.

Imaging Findings

Anteroposterior view of the pelvis was normal (Fig. 3.9), and although frog-leg views demonstrated a slipped capital upper femoral epiphysis (arrow) in the left hip (Fig. 3.10), it was reported as normal.

Due to persistent pain, new radiographs of the knee and hip were performed, which were also reported as normal.

The patient returned to the emergency room with persisting pain. On clinical examination, she described the fluctuating hip, outer thigh, and knee pain to have had a spontaneous onset without prior trauma or extra efforts. The pain increased at the beginning of activity. It decreased as the activity progressed, with rest and while sitting. There was no fever in this period. Patient's pain showed moderate improvement with ibuprofen. She showed no other symptoms.

An ultrasound study (Fig. 3.11) detected a hip joint effusion (arrow).

With the suspicion of early Perthes disease, an MRI (T1-weighted coronal MR image) was performed (Fig. 3.12) showing widening of the left femoral physis (arrow), with minimal displacement, bone edema, and a joint effusion. A definitive diagnosis of proximal femur epiphysiolysis was made.

She underwent osteosynthesis with cannulated screws.

Case 3.4: Proximal Tibia Epiphysiolysis with Posterior Metaphyseal Fracture (Salter-Harris Type II)

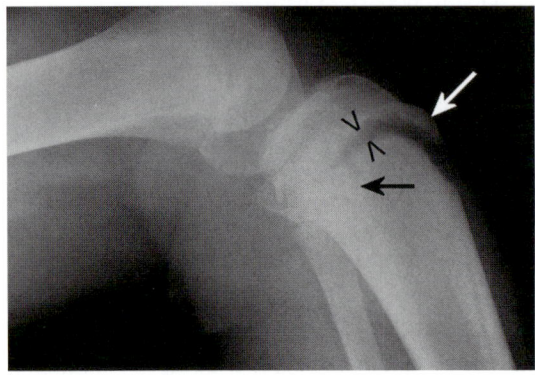

Fig. 3.13

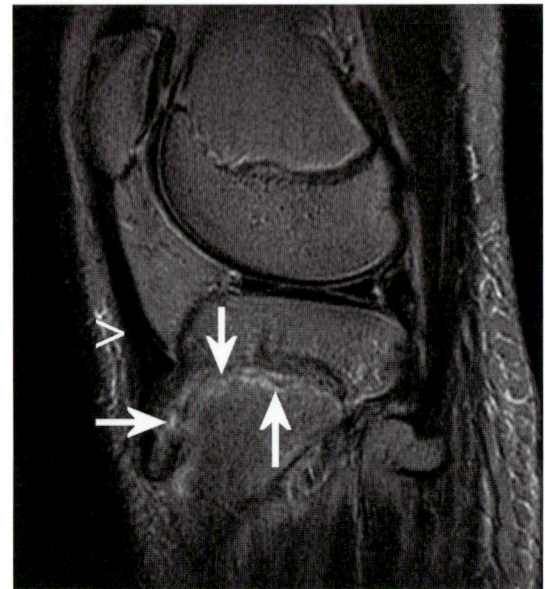

Fig. 3.14

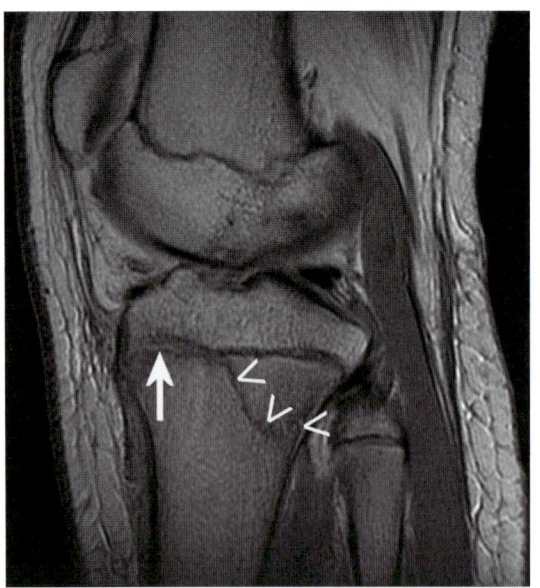

Fig. 3.15

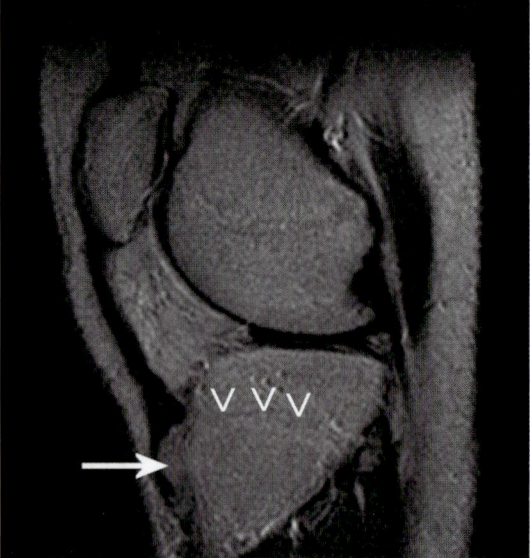

Fig. 3.16

A 16-year-old basketball player complained of acute knee pain and movement restriction after jumping.

Comments

Proximal tibial fractures are not common in children. Proximal tibial conform about 1 % of all epiphysiolyses. Physeal fractures and tibial spine or tibial tubercle (TT) avulsions are more common in older children and adolescents and, in developed countries, are usually related to sports activity. The epiphyseal plate consists of several layers: reserve, immature, and mature proliferative-germinal layers and hypertrophic and calcification layers. The germinal layers are more attached to the epiphyseal bone; therefore, the physis rupture is easier at the metaphysical side and carries a lesser risk of growth disturbance (Salter-Harris types I and II). The proximal tibial epiphyseal plate closure is asymmetric, from posterior to anterior. Thus, in adolescents, the anterior part is weaker than the posterior one (more calcified). In basketball players, hurdlers, high jumpers, or gymnasts, for example, a quadriceps femoris sharp contraction to boost the jump may cause the anterior tibial epiphysiolysis (including anterior tibial tubercle). The patient failing to keep knee extension and landing with a flexed knee can cause the posterior metaphyseal fracture (Salter-Harris type II): Böhler's injury mechanism "leap with a bad landing." Another possible mechanism of injury is related to forced flexion against actively contracting quadriceps on landing after jumping. Patients present with pain, swelling, and deformity at the anteroinferior part of the knee, proximal patellar displacement, and quadriceps spasm. They are unable to move the knee or walk. The first author who classified the

TT avulsion fracture by the fragment's size was Watson Jones. Ogden described subtypes regarding intra-articular extension and TT comminution. However, Ryu in 1985 was the first to describe its association with a posterior metaphyseal fracture (type IV) (as seen in this case). Displaced fractures or intra-articular extension merit prompts referral to assess the need for osteosynthesis (Ogden IB, II, III). Little or undisplaced TT fractures (Ogden IA) can be treated nonsurgically: reduction and knee immobilization with a long-leg cast, as was this patient. Patients should be advised against returning to full sporting activity until they have regained 80–90 % of the quadriceps strength of the unaffected side.

Imaging Findings

Lateral radiograph (Fig. 3.13) shows proximal tibial anterior epiphysiolysis (arrowheads), with tibial tubercle (white arrow) extension. The posterior metaphyseal fracture (black arrow) is hardly seen. The flexed position is due to the patient's inability for extending the knee.

Sagittal T2 spin-echo-weighted image shows good reduction of the epiphysiolysis and tibial tubercle avulsion with some residual edema (hyperintense signal) (arrows). No patella tendon tear (arrowhead) (Fig. 3.14) is seen.

Sagittal proton density spin-echo-weighted image shows the undisplaced thin posterior metaphyseal fracture (arrowheads) and the reduced anterior epiphysiolysis (arrow). No meniscus tear (Fig. 3.15) is seen.

Final sagittal T2 spin-echo-weighted image shows complete consolidation of the tibial tubercle (arrow) epiphysiolysis (arrowheads) without growth bone complication (Fig. 3.16).

Case 3.5: Traumatic Distal Femoral Bone Infarct

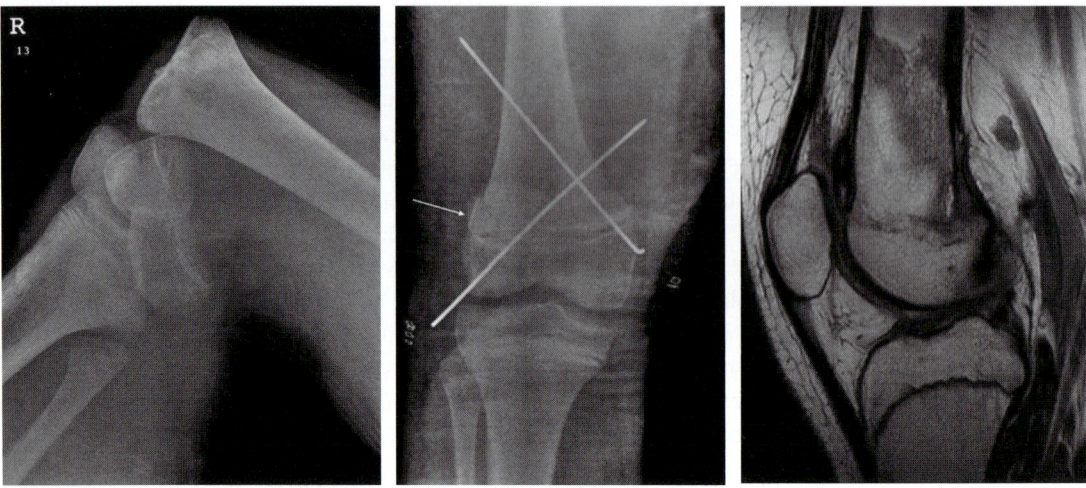

Fig. 3.17   Fig. 3.18   Fig. 3.19

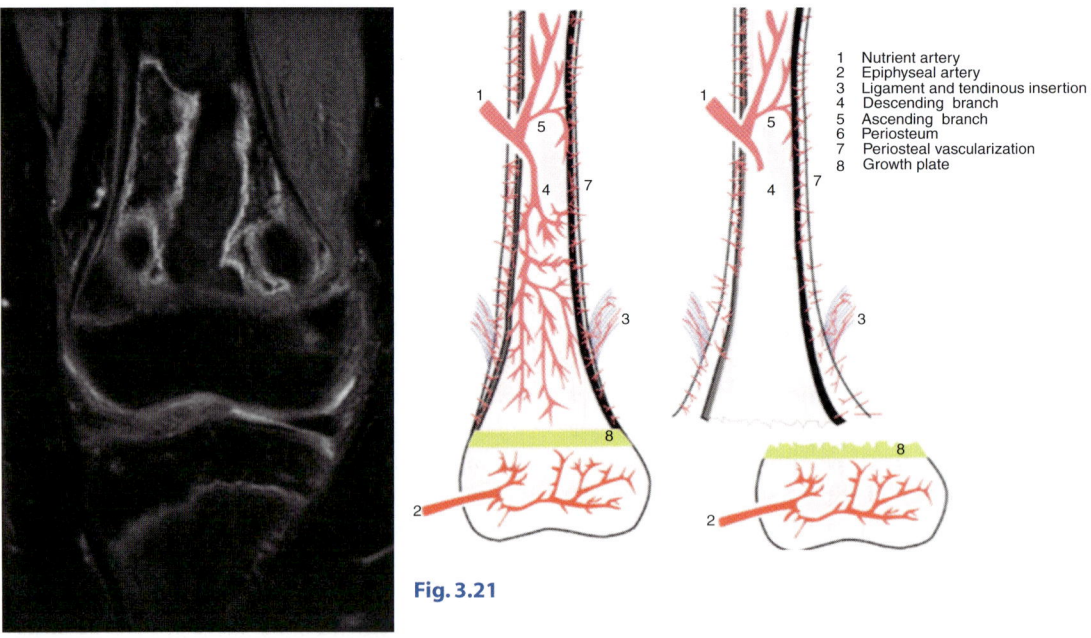

Fig. 3.20

Fig. 3.21

1   Nutrient artery
2   Epiphyseal artery
3   Ligament and tendinous insertion
4   Descending branch
5   Ascending branch
6   Periosteum
7   Periosteal vascularization
8   Growth plate

A 14-year-old boy suffered a motocross accident. Physical examination showed significant right knee deformity and swelling, without distal neurovascular involvement.

Comments

Bone infarcts are due to vascular disorders. They are usually seen in the long bones' metaphyseal regions, associated to underlying systemic conditions, such as sickle cell disease, lupus erythematosus, acute lymphocytic leukemia, non-Hodgkin lymphoma, and renal transplantation. Nevertheless, they can also be seen in the absence of related medical disease. Although rare, they can be found after a high-energy injury.

A suspected bone infarct diagnosis is not difficult on plain radiographs on the basis of its characteristic serpiginous appearance. However, diagnostic confirmation is not so easy, and differentiation with osteomyelitis and malignancy is mandatory.

MR findings of bone infarct are very characteristic, with a serpentine rim that corresponds to the reactive sclerosis seen on plain radiographs. In acute and subacute stages, the central infarct is equal to normal medullar fat signal and corresponds to avascular bone tissue. On MRI, both T1- and T2-weighted sequences show a thin, low-signal rim with a typical serpentine border. All these medullary changes are not seen on plain films, probably due to circumferential periosteal thickening. The reactive osteoblastic tissue implicated in peripheral bone consolidation and remodelation is responsible for this low T1 signal. T2-weighted fat-suppression images show peripherically bright serpiginous lesions due to edema. This set of characteristic MR findings can lead to the bone infarct diagnosis.

Long bones have three arterial inputs: (1) nutrient artery, (2) periosteal arteries, and (3) epiphyseal arteries (Fig. 3.21). Their main supply is through the nutrient artery.

Anastomoses between the nutrient and periosteal system can develop in response to injury. Damage to both nutrient and metaphyseal supply of the growing distal femur can result in marrow necrosis.

Long vascular anatomy in children differs from that in adults. The epiphyseal and metaphyseal vascular supply are independent of each other between ages 1 and 16. Distal metaphyseal trabecular bone vascularization depends on terminal branches from the nutrient artery and metaphyseal circulation. Epiphyseal supply, however, depends just on the epiphyseal artery. The barrier between both vascularization systems is the growth plate. Growth plate closure at about age 16 allows continuity between both systems.

This case's high-energy injury caused serious damage on the nutrient and periosteal arterial systems, with preservation of the epiphyseal vascular supply. The thick periosteal reaction indicates that the small periosteal arteries were preserved and were able to supply most of the metaphyseal cortex, but not the marrow cavity. This periosteal response is responsible for the false epiphyseal osteoporosis appearance on plain radiographs.

Radiological Findings

Plain radiographs show a type II Salter-Harris physeal injury, with a lateral Thurston-Holland fragment (arrow). Closed reduction was performed under general anesthesia and fluoroscope imaging (Figs. 3.17 and 3.18).

Three months after injury, T1-weighted MR images showed a thin, low-signal rim with a typical serpentine border, corresponding to reactive sclerosis (Fig. 3.19). On a fat-suppressed T2-weighted image, the center of this lesion showed the same signal as medullar fatty tissue (Fig. 3.20) and indicating avascular bone tissue. These characteristic MR findings led us to the bone infarct diagnosis.

Case 3.6: Triplane Fracture of the Distal Tibia

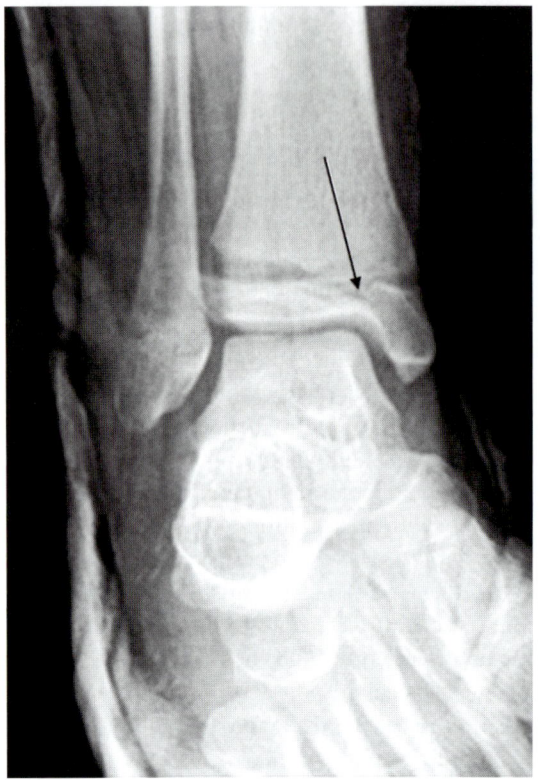

Fig. 3.22

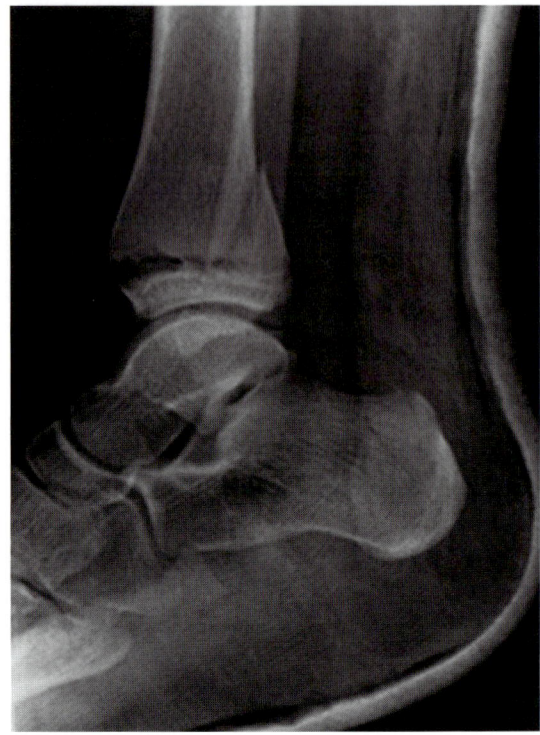

Fig. 3.23

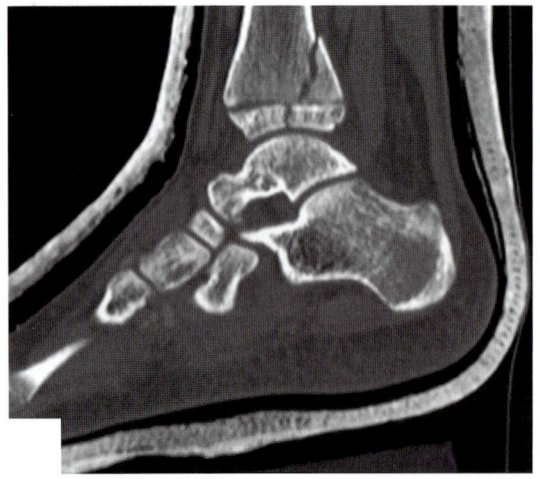

Fig. 3.24

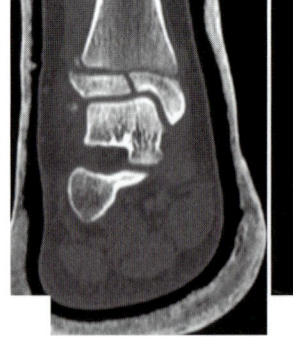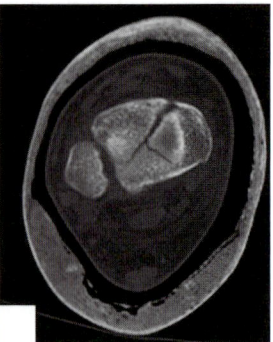

Fig. 3.25

An 11-year-old child had this ankle fracture after an external rotation injury while playing soccer.

Comment

Triplane fractures represent 5–10 % of pediatric intra-articular ankle injuries and typically occur in children aged 12–15. Most epiphyseal fractures of the ankle can be classified according to Salter and Harris, but an appreciable number do not follow that scheme. Triplane fractures of the distal tibia are multiplanar injuries:

1. Coronal. Fracture through the distal tibial metaphysis, in its posterior part. In the lateral radiograph, it appears as a type II or IV Salter-Harris injury.
2. Transverse. Epiphysiolysis through the anterior and lateral parts of the physis.
3. Sagittal. Fracture through the distal epiphysis. In the anteroposterior radiograph, it simulates a type III epiphysiolysis.

Triplane fractures can be classified in type I (two-part fractures) and type II/III (three-part fracture).

Diagnosis of the triplane fracture on *radiographs* can be difficult. Computed tomography must be performed.

Computed tomography and three-dimensional reconstructions improve understanding of injury patterns and assist in management decision.

MR imaging is generally used for detecting post-injury complications, such as bony bridging and growth arrest.

Undisplaced triplane fractures can be treated with immobilization in a long-leg cast. Displaced fractures can be treated with closed or open reduction and internal fixation through an antero-lateral or anteromedial approach.

Radiological Findings

Anteroposterior radiography of the right ankle (Fig. 3.22) shows a Salter-Harris type III epiphyseal fracture. Lateral radiography (Fig. 3.23) and sagittal CT (Fig. 3.24) show a Salter-Harris type II injury. Coronal CT imaging (Fig. 3.25 left) shows also a Salter-Harris type III epiphyseal fracture. The axial CT (Fig. 3.25. right) shows the "Mercedes-Benz star" fracture configuration.

Case 3.7: Monteggia Fracture-Dislocation Associated with Ulna Plastic Bowing

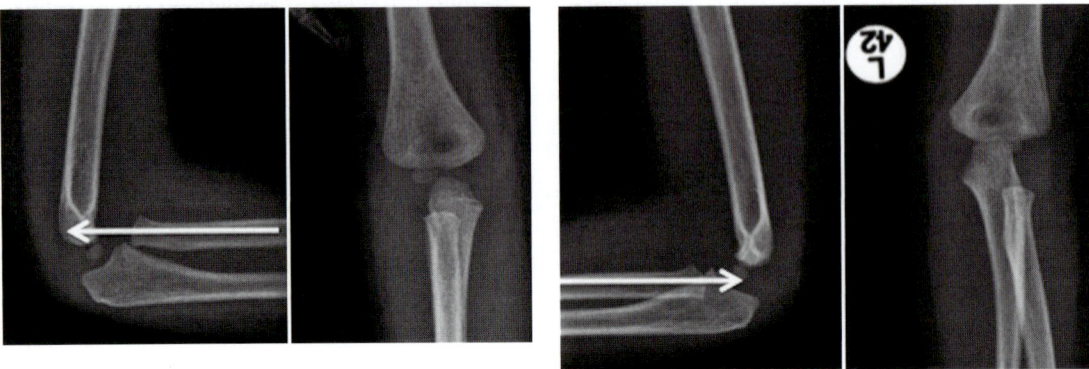

Fig. 3.26

Fig. 3.27

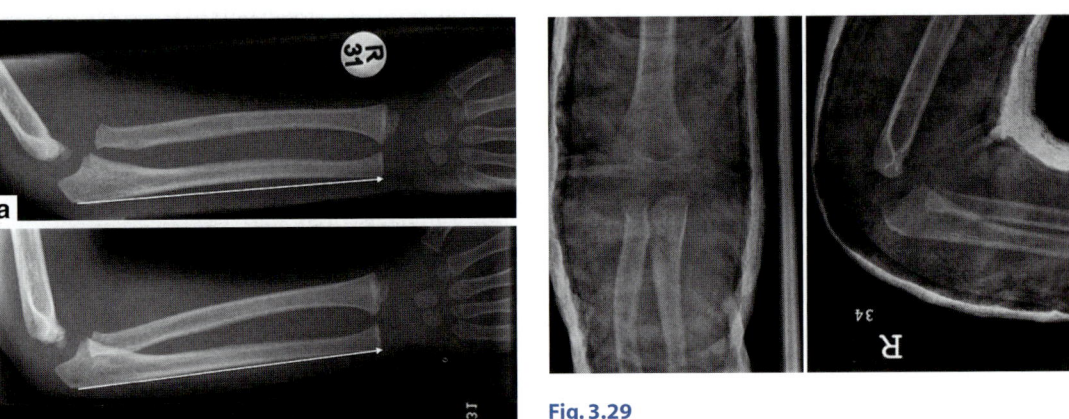

Fig. 3.28

Fig. 3.29

A 4-year-old child fell from a 1-m height injuring his right forearm.

Comment

Peri-elbow fractures are the most common in children, but they can also be some of the most elusive to detect.

Giovanni Battista Monteggia described the first two of what would become known as *Monteggia fractures* in 1814. They account for approximately 1–2 % of all forearm fractures, and they generally refer to a proximal ulnar fracture with an associated radial head dislocation.

Although clinical presentation may be suggestive of a Monteggia fracture, the diagnosis is most often confirmed by plain radiography.

Anteroposterior and lateral forearm views should be acquired to evaluate the radiocapitellar, radioulnar, and radiohumeral joints plus radial and ulnar shafts for evidence of fractures or dislocations.

The vast majority of elbow fractures are accompanied by fluid within the elbow joint. An elbow joint effusion is easily detected on well-positioned lateral views. It is seen as anterior and posterior displacement of distal humeral fat pads. The anterior fat pad is the sum of radial and coronoid fat pads, normally pressed into the shallow radial and coronoid fossa by the brachialis muscle. On a lateral radiograph with the elbow at 90° flexion, the anterior fat pad is normally seen as a faint radiolucent line parallel to the anterior distal humerus. The posterior fat pad is normally pressed into the deep olecranon fossae by the triceps tendon and is invisible on a true lateral radiograph.

To diagnose a radial head dislocation, a line can be drawn through the radial shaft extending through the radial head using an elbow radiograph. If the radial head is in its normal anatomical position, the line should penetrate the capitellum in all radiographic views, especially the lateral ones.

Particular attention should be paid to the ulnar appearance, especially for signs of plastic deformation or other pathology.

In the pediatric population, early identification and conservative management have been shown to correlate with good result. Nevertheless, there is no standard treatment protocol and several authors have advised more aggressive surgical management of this injury.

Imaging Findings

Anteroposterior and lateral right elbow radiographs (Fig. 3.26) show a Monteggia fracture. A white line is drawn through the radial shaft passing above the capitellum (arrowhead) indicating an anterior dislocation of the radial head. The contralateral radiographs show the normal position (Fig. 3.27).

Comparing plain lateral forearm and elbow films of both arms (Fig. 3.28), the radial head dislocation and acute plastic bowing of the ulna are seen in the right (above), while the normal left side is shown below. Plastic deformation refers to bending or bowing without a fracture as a result of the reduced mineral content in pediatric cortical bone.

Manipulated under general anesthesia, successful repositioning of the dislocated radial head and correction of ulnar bowing were achieved. Postoperative anteroposterior and lateral radiographs of the right elbow show the normal position of the radial head (Fig. 3.29).

Case 3.8: Supracondylar Humerus Fracture with Associated Arterial Spasm

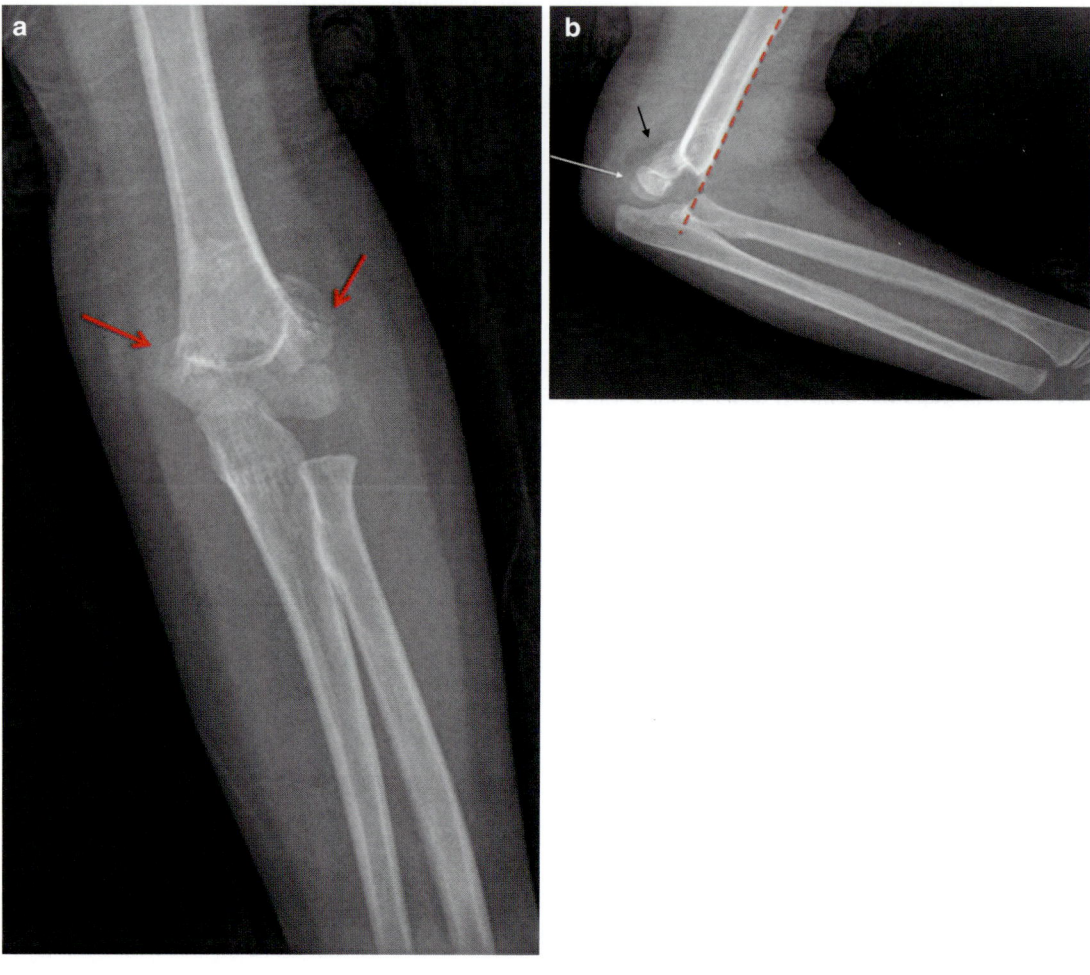

Fig. 3.30

A 6-year-old boy fell from a bicycle onto his extended arm. On arrival to the emergency room, he was in great pain and presented severe functional impotence.

Comments

Among the distal humeral fractures in children, supracondylar is the most common accounting for about 60 % of all elbow fractures.

Most of these occur in children younger than 10 and usually between the ages 5 and 8. Predisposing conditions are increased collateral ligament looseness, bone immaturity, and the specific relationship of bone structures in the elbow joint.

More than 95 % of supracondylar fractures follow a hyperextension mechanism due to falling on an outstretched hand. The elbow locks in hyperextension, so the olecranon is pushed into the fossa causing the anterior humeral cortex to bend and eventually break. If the force continues, both the anterior and posterior cortices will fracture.

The Gartland classification (1959) is the most commonly used: radiographic analysis provides guidance in selecting treatment options. It divides fractures in:

- *Type I*: often difficult to see on x-rays since there is only minimal displacement. Most of these are greenstick or torus fractures. The only diagnostic clue may be a positive fat pad sign. These patients are treated with casting.
- In *Type II fractures*, there is displacement but the posterior cortex is intact. These fractures require closed reduction.
- *Type III fractures* are completely dislocated and are at risk for malunion and neurovascular complications. They require closed or, if necessary, open reduction.

Malunion will result in the classic "gunstock" deformity due to rotation or inadequate correction of medial collapse. Posterolateral displacement of the distal fragment can be associated to neurovascular bundle injury by displacing it over the medial metaphyseal spike. Nerve injuries almost always result in neuropraxis that tends to resolve in 3–4 months.

Radiological Findings

Anteroposterior radiographs show posterior displacement of humeral condyles (Fig. 3.30a). Baumann's angle is obtained by measuring the angle between a line perpendicular to the

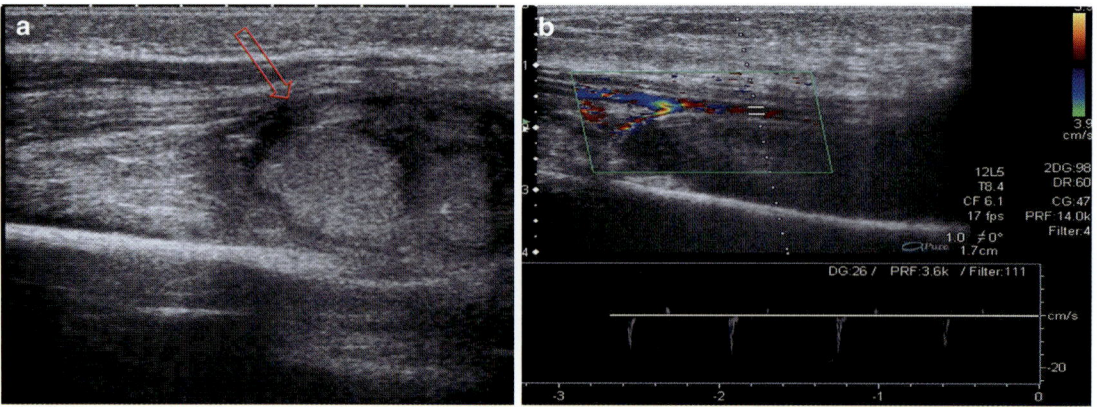

Fig. 3.31

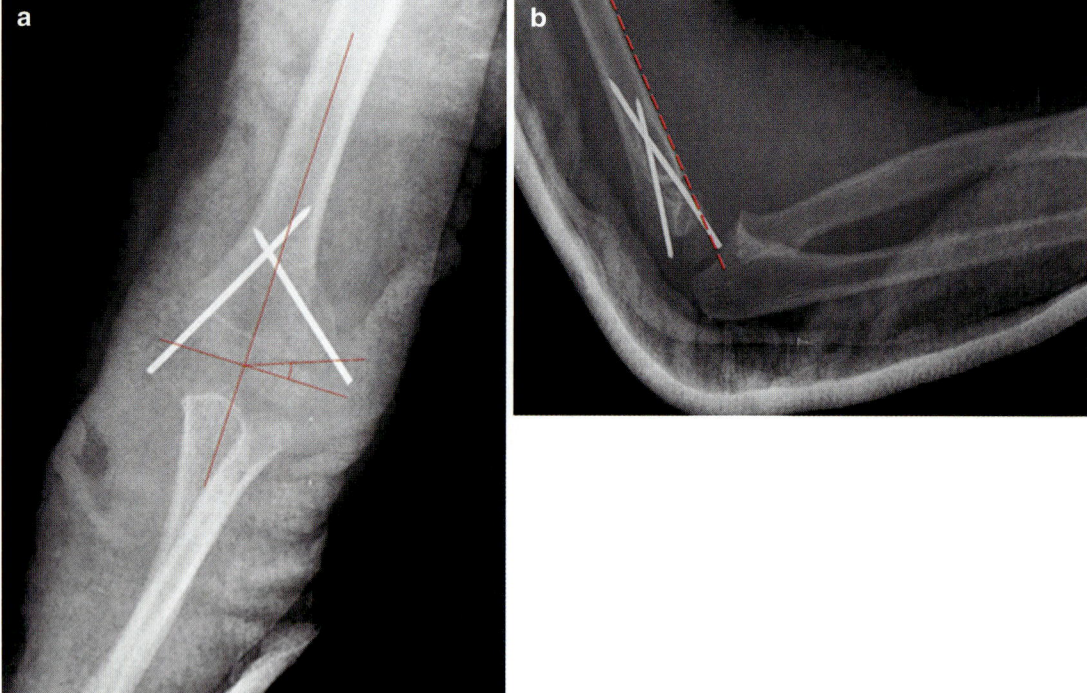

Fig. 3.32

humeral longitudinal axis and another line parallel to the capitellum growth plate (Fig. 3.32a). It is commonly used to evaluate distal humeral and elbow varus/valgus deviation after reduction. It varies among individuals; therefore, exploring the contralateral elbow could be necessary.

A lateral x-ray shows fat pad displacement (black arrow) due to the intra-articular hematoma derived from the fracture (Fig. 3.30b). Posterior capitellum displacement (white arrow) beyond the anterior humeral line is also observed. The anterior humeral line (AHL) measured on the lateral plain film (Fig. 3.30b) represents a longitudinal line running from the humeral diaphysis' edge. It normally passes through the capitellum's middle-third.

The present case was diagnosed as a Gartland type 3 supracondylar fracture. A Doppler ultrasound was performed due to the radial artery's low pulse noticed during the examination. A 5 cm hematoma was observed at the elbow flexure (Fig. 3.31a) causing arterial spasm without vascular laceration (Fig. 3.31b).

After reduction and K-wire fixation, adequate position of the humerus capitellum can be observed on both the anteroposterior and lateral x-ray films (Figs. 3.32a, b).

Case 3.9: Greenstick Fracture

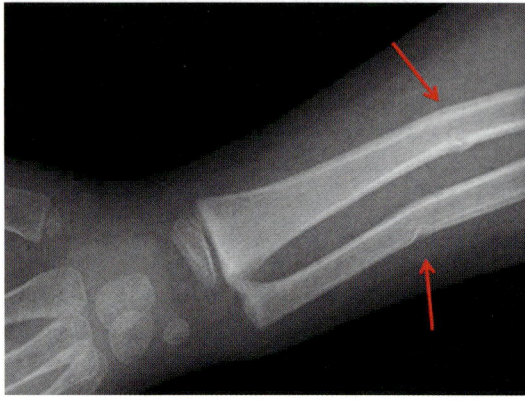

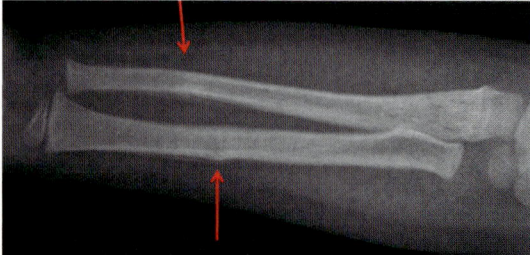

Fig. 3.34

Fig. 3.33

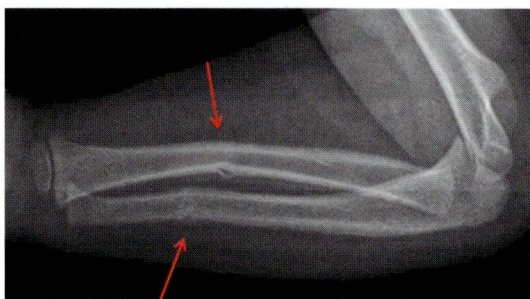

Fig. 3.35

A 3-year-old boy fell while running in the park and hit his right forearm on a rock.

Comments

A greenstick fracture is defined as a one in which the cortex is completely disrupted on the bone convexity and incompletely on the concave aspect. It is named by analogy to green wood, which similarly breaks on the outside when bent.

They usually occur in children and teens as their immature, relatively soft, and flexible bones are covered by a thick, fibrous periosteum layer. The adult's bones are more brittle and also surrounded by a thinner and less restrictive periosteum, so they tend to break.

Forces lateral to the bone may cause only one cortex to break, while the other cortex only bends. The greenstick fracture pattern is consequence of bending forces.

Physeal injuries occur frequently during the preadolescent growth spurt, when there is a transient cortical porosity caused by increased in calcium requirements and bone turnover.

Basic forms of greenstick fracture are:
- Type 1: Cortical transverse fracture extending into the bone's midportion along its longitudinal axis without disrupting the opposite cortex
- Type 2 (torus or buckling fracture): compression bony failure without cortical disruption on the tension side
- Type 3: bow fracture in which the bone becomes curved along its longitudinal axis

Greenstick fractures are stable since part of the bone remains intact and unbroken. Thus, this type of fracture normally causes a bend to the injured body part, rather than a distinct deformity, which is problematic for diagnosis. These kinds of fractures are usually associated with volar and supination deformities.

Although non-accidental injuries more commonly cause spiral fractures, a blow on the forearm or shin could also cause greenstick fractures.

The standard treatment of impacted greenstick fractures of the distal forearm in children younger than 13 is cast immobilization for 2–4 weeks. Surgery is only necessary if instability, soft tissue interposition, or compartment syndrome are present.

Imaging Findings

Distal radius and ulna type 1–2 greenstick fracture radiographs show the posteromedial cortical disruption of both the ulna and radius (Figs. 3.33, 3.34, and 3.35) with some degree of radial impaction and bending. Only one side of the cortex is disrupted, whereas the other is merely bent with no interruption. Notice the discrete cortical swelling or interruption seen on both views but best on the lateral film (Fig. 3.34).

Case 3.10: Tillaux Fracture and Grade 4 Epiphysiolysis in Salter-Harris Classification

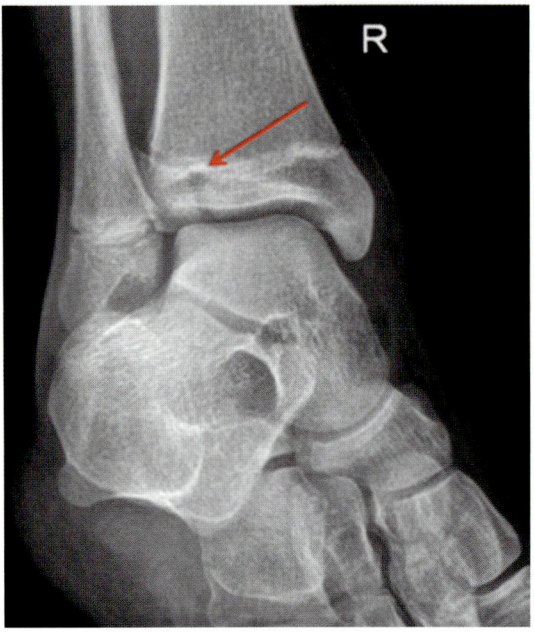

Fig. 3.36

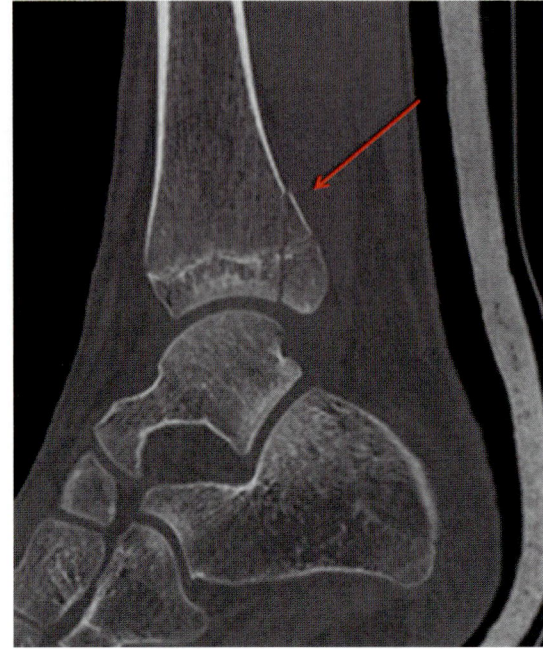

Fig. 3.37

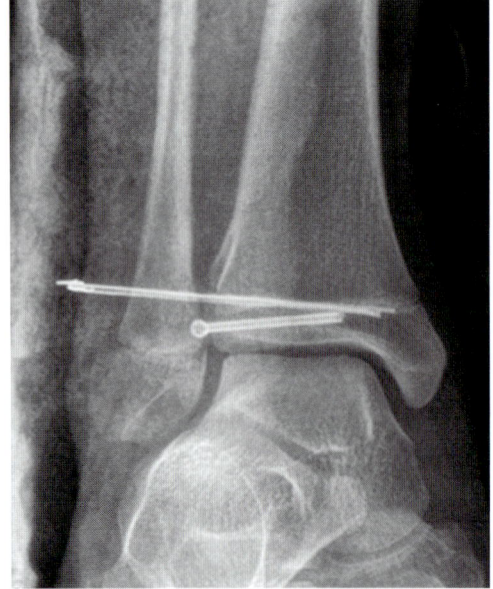

Fig. 3.38

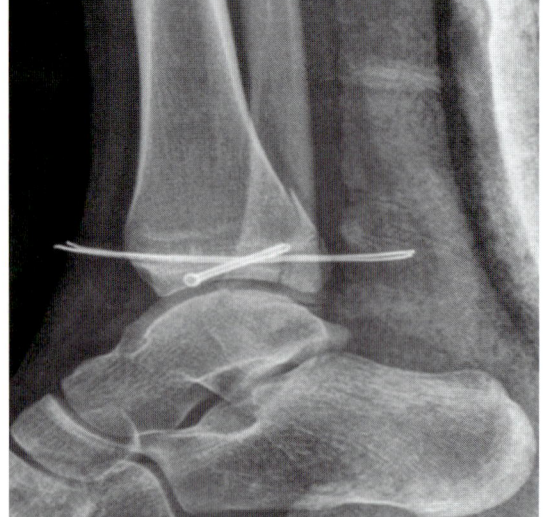

Fig. 3.39

A 12-year-old girl without relevant medical history injured her right ankle while skateboarding, due to external rotation of the leg.

Comments

Tillaux fractures correspond to Salter and Harris type III and involve the anterolateral portion of the tibial epiphysis. They are intra-articular. The fracture line extends vertically from the tibial distal articular surface upwards to the lateral cortex. The fragment is roughly quadrangular in shape.

Tillaux fracture can develop due to the lateral growth plate's weakness. It occurs in adolescents, after the epiphyseal plate's middle and medial parts close but before the lateral part does so is closed (usually around ages 12–15). This allows for an avulsion fracture at the anterior tibiofibular ligament's attachment point. In adults, these lesions are not common since the tibiofibular ligament tends to get disrupted before the bone breaks.

In an external rotation force setting, Tillaux and triplane fractures can occur. They, as with other Salter-Harris growth plate injuries, do not fit strictly into any classification scheme and are not easily evaluated on plain radiographs. Further lateral rotation displaces the fracture and may be associated to a lateral malleolar fracture.

The present case shows a Tillaux fracture associated to a Salter-Harris grade 4 epiphysiolysis in the posterior tibial distal epiphysial region. These findings are analogous to triplane fractures but with two different fracture lines.

Treatment consists in reduction and fixation if the fracture displacement is equal or greater than 2 mm.

Imaging Findings

Preoperative radiographs showed a Tillaux fracture with a lateral epiphyseal plate displacement of more than 2 mm in the anteroposterior (AP) view (Fig. 3.36). A computed tomography scan sagittal reconstruction demonstrates a grade 4 epiphysiolysis in the posterior region of the distal tibia (Fig. 3.37). Figures 3.38 and 3.39 depict the postoperative radiograph after open reduction and fixation with a screw and a percutaneous Kirschner wire.

Further Reading

Books

Canale ST (2008) Fractures and dislocation in children. In: Canale ST, Beaty JH (eds) Campbell's operative orthopedics, 11th edn. Elseviers Science, Philadelphia

DeLee JC, Drez D Jr, Miller MD (eds) (2003) DeLee and Drez's orthopaedic sports medicine, 2nd edn. Elseviers Science, Philadelphia

Martino F, Defilippi C, Caudana R (eds) (2011) Imaging of pediatric bone and joint trauma. Springer, Milan

Ogden JA (ed) (1990) Skeletal injury in the child, 2nd edn. WB Saunders, Philadelphia

Resnick D (2002) Diagnosis of bone and joint disorders, 4th edn. WB Saunders, Philadelphia

Websites

Clinique du Sport, Bordeaux. http://www.image-echo graphie.net/

http://www.radiologyassistant.nl

http://www.radiologyeducation.com/

Skeletal Trauma Radiology. http://www.med-ed.virginia. edu/courses/rad/ext/

Wheeles textbook of Orthopaedics. http://www.wheeles-sonline.com/

Articles

Bhatnagar R, Nzegwu NI, Miller NH (2006) Diagnosis and treatment of common fractures in children femoral shaft fractures and supracondylar humeral fractures. J Surg Orthop Adv 15(1):1–15

Britton PD (1988) Adolescent-type Tillaux fracture of the ankle: two case reports. Arch Emerg Med 5(3): 180–183

Brubacher JW, Dodds SD (2008) Pediatric supracondylar fractures of the distal humerus. Curr Rev Musculoskelet Med 1(3–4):190–196

Chasm RM, Swencki SA (2010) Pediatric orthopedic emergencies. Emerg Med Clin North Am 28:907–926

Ghanem I, Karam JA, Widmann RF (2011) Surgical epiphysiodesis indications and techniques: update. Curr Opin Pediatr 23(1):53–59

Gholson JJ, Bae DS, Zurakowski D et al (2011) Scaphoid fractures in children and adolescents: contemporary injury patterns and factors influencing time to union. J Bone Joint Surg Am 93:1210–1219

Huckstadt T, Klitscher D, Weltzien A, Müller LP, Rommens PR, Schier F (2007) Pediatrics fracture of the carpal scaphoid. A retrospective clinical and radiological study. J Pediatr Orthop 27:447–450

Johnson EO, Soultanis K, Soucacos PN (2004) Vascular anatomy and microcirculation of skeletal zones vulnerable to osteonecrosis: vascularization of the femoral head. Orthop Clin North Am 35:285–291

Kim JR, Song KH, Song KJ, Lee HS (2010) Treatment outcomes of triplane and Tillaux fractures of the ankle in adolescence. Clin Orthop Surg 2(1):34–38

Kocher MS, Tucker R (2006) Pediatric athlete hip disorders. Clin Sports Med 25:241–253

Lalandle K, Letts M (2005) Traumatic growth arrest of the distal tibia: a clinical and radiographic review. Can J Surg 2:143–147

Loder RT (2006) Controversies in slipped capital femoral epiphysis. Orthop Clin North Am 37:211–221

Magnano GM, Lucigrai G, De Filippi C (1998) Diagnosis imaging of the early slipped capital femoral epiphysis. Radiol Med (Torino) 95:16–20

Mangwani J, Nadarajah R, Paterson JM (2006) Supracondylar humeral fractures in children: ten years' experience in a teaching hospital. J Bone Joint Surg Br 88(3):362–365

Masquijo JJ, Willis BR (2010) Scaphoid nonunions in children and adolescents. Surgical treatment with bone grafting and internal fixation. J Pediatr Orthop 30:119–124

Munk PL, Helms CA, Holt RG (1989) Immature bone infarcts: findings on plain radiographs and MR scans. AJR Am J Roentgenol 152(3):547–549

Nanno M, Takuya S, Ito H (2007) Three cases of pediatric Monteggia fracture-dislocation associated with acute plastic bowing of the ulna. Am J Orthop (Belle Mead NJ) 36(5):E80–E82

Pannier S, Odent T, Milet A et al (2006) Tillaux fractures in teenagers: a review of nineteen cases. Rev Chir Orthop Reparatrice Appar Mot 92(2):158–164

Randsborg PH, Sivertsen EA (2012) Classification of distal radius fractures in children: good inter- and intraobserver reliability, which improves with clinical experience. BMC Musculoskelet Disord 13:6

Rapariz JM, Ocete G, Gonzalez-Herranz P, López-Mondejar JA, Domenech J, Burgos J, Amaya S (1996) Distal tibial triplane fractures: long-term follow-up. J Pediatr Orthop 16(1):113–118

Ryu RK, Debenham JO (1985) An unusual avulsion fracture of the proximal tibial epiphysis. Case report and proposed addition to the Watson-Jones classification. Clin Orthop 194:181–184

Salter RB, Harris WR (1963) Injuries involving the epiphyseal Plate. J Bone Joint Surg Am 45:587–622

Schurz M, Binder H, Platzer P, Schulz M, Hajdu S, Vécsei V (2010) Physeal injuries of the distal tibia: long-term results in 376 patients. Int Orthop 34(4):547–552

Shelton WR, Canale ST (1979) Fractures of the tibia through the proximal tibial epiphyseal. J Bone Joint Surg Am 61:167–173

Stefanich RJ, Lozman J (1986) The juvenile fracture of tillaux. Clin Orthop Relat Res 210:219–227

Overuse Injuries

4

Rosa Mónica Rodrigo, Joan C. Vilanova,
Maria Jose Ereño, and Juan María Santisteban

Contents

R.M. Rodrigo (✉)
Department of Radiology,
Resonancia Magnética Bilbao, Bilbao, Spain
e-mail: rmrodrigo@resonanciamagnetica.com

J.C. Vilanova
Department of Radiology, Clínica Girona-Hospital
Sta. Caterina, University of Girona, Girona, Spain

M.J. Ereño
Department of Radiology, Resonancia Magnética
Bilbao, Bilbao, Spain

Department of Radiology, Hospital de Galdakano,
Vizcaya, Spain

J.M. Santisteban
Medical Services, Athletic Club Bilbao, Bilbao,
Spain

Department of Physiology, Faculty of Medicine
and Odontology, University of the Basque Country,
Bilbao, Spain

R.M. Rodrigo et al., *Sports Injuries in Children and Adolescents*,
DOI 10.1007/978-3-642-54746-1_4, © Springer-Verlag Berlin Heidelberg 2014

Case 4.1: Juvenile Kyphosis (Type II) or Atypical Scheuermann's Disease

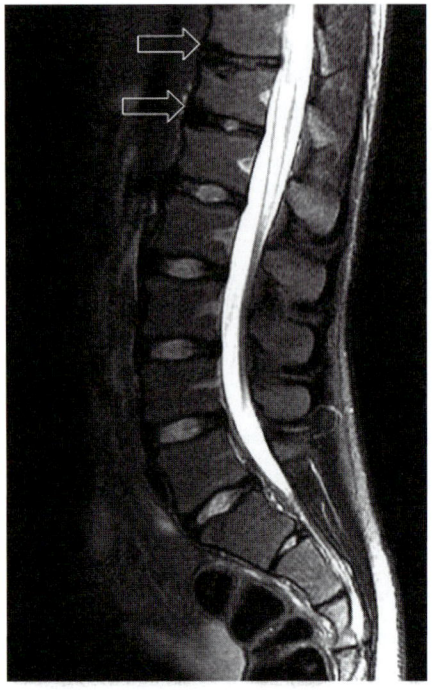

Fig. 4.1

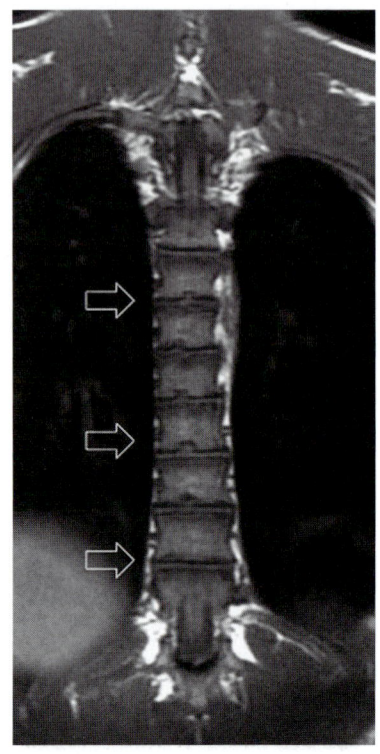

Fig. 4.2

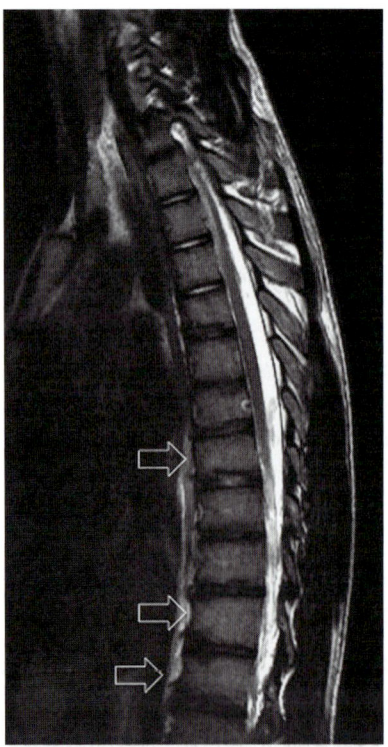

Fig. 4.3

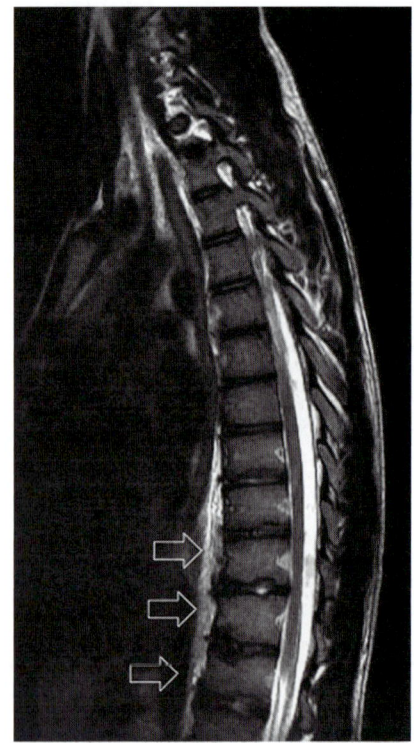

Fig. 4.4

A 14-year-old male soccer player complained of pain along the thoracolumbar spine which had increased with hyperextension maneuvers. Spondylolysis was initially suspected so an MRI of the lumbar area was performed. Image findings indicated a new study of the thoracic spine.

Comments

Osteochondrosis is a family of joint orthopedic diseases occurring in children and adolescents. Scheuermann's disease is considered a form of spinal juvenile osteochondrosis. It consists of a thoracic/thoracolumbar hyperkyphosis due to wedged vertebrae.

The true incidence of juvenile kyphosis is not known and ranges between 1 and 8 %. The exact etiology is unknown. It has a genetic background and develops due to an ossification disturbance of the vertebral bodies. The front of the upper spine does not grow as fast as the back, so that vertebrae become wedge shaped, with the narrow part of the wedge towards the front.

Pain can arise from postural changes. Cervical and lumbar pain is caused by compensatory hyperlordosis above or below the primary deformity.

There are two types with different diagnostic criteria:

1. Juvenile kyphosis (type I) or "classic" Scheuermann's disease
   (a) Wedging of more than 5° in one or more vertebrae in the thoracic or thoracolumbar region
   (b) Disk space narrowing
   (c) End plate irregularities
   (d) Increased thoracic or thoracolumbar kyphosis
       Schmorl's nodes are often associated with juvenile kyphosis but are not a pathognomonic sign.
2. Juvenile kyphosis (type II, "lumbar") or atypical Scheuermann's disease
Obligatory criteria:
   (a) End plate irregularities in one or several vertebral bodies of the lumbar or thoracolumbar area
   (b) Increased sagittal diameter of vertebral bodies (without significant wedging), loss of lumbar lordosis
   (c) Disk space narrowing
Possible criteria:
   (d) Apophyseal separation
   (e) Schmorl's nodes

Back pain occurs mainly during the day and under loading and is more common in Type II. This atypical Scheuermann's disease is commonly seen in athletes as a consequence of mechanical overloading.

Idiopathic thoracic hyperkyphosis ("round-back," "poor posture") must be differentiated from juvenile kyphosis: clinically, postural thoracic hyperkyphosis is mobile, more harmonic, and not as localized as Scheuermann's kyphosis. On radiographs, there is no wedge deformation, and disk space height is not decreased. Usually, the deformity corrects on extension.

The definitive diagnosis of juvenile kyphosis can often be made by conventional radiographs alone. However, MRI highlights end plate abnormalities, premature disk degeneration, and vertebral wedging significantly better.

Treatment largely depends on the degree of kyphosis. This soccer player was treated without a brace with physical therapy, mobilization, and strengthening exercises.

Radiological Findings

Sagittal MR FSE T2-weighted image of the lumbar spine (Fig. 4.1) does not reveal pathological findings for spondylolysis. Some irregularities are seen in several vertebral end plates of lower thoracic vertebrae (open arrows). Coronal FSE T1-weighted image (Fig. 4.2) and sagittal FSE T2-weighted images (Figs. 4.3 and 4.4) of the thoracic spine show vertebral end plate irregularities in the T6–T12 segment, slight increase in sagittal diameter of vertebral bodies, disk space narrowing, and normal lumbar lordosis, which are typical of juvenile kyphosis (type II).

Case 4.2: Osteochondrosis of the Apophysis of the Base of the Fifth Metatarsal or Iselin Disease

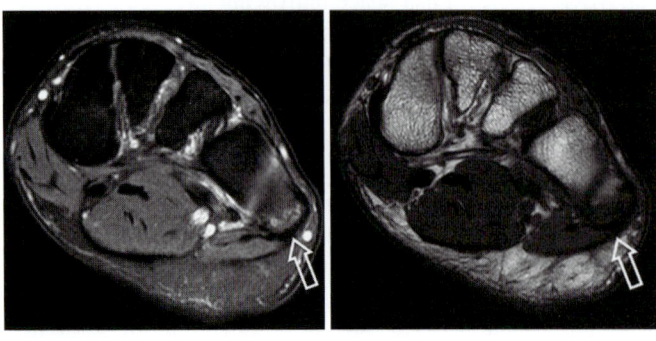

Fig. 4.5

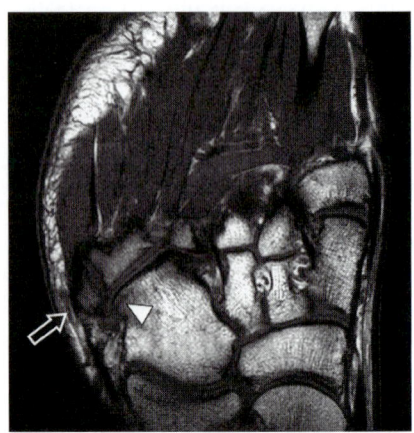

Fig. 4.6

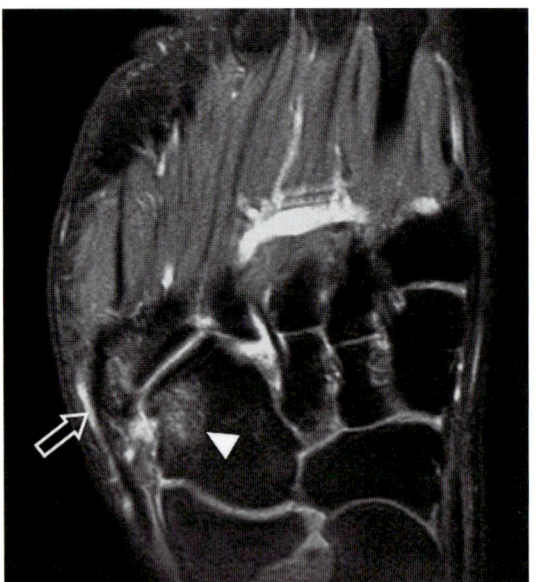

Fig. 4.7

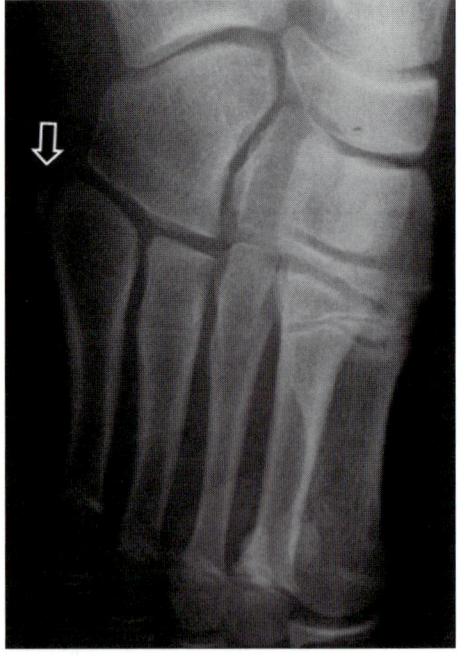

Fig. 4.8

A 16-year-old soccer player presented with localized pain on the lateral aspect of the left foot while training.

Comments

The proximal fifth metatarsal is the insertion site of three ligaments (lateral band of the plantar fascia and plantar and dorsal fourth to fifth metatarsal ligaments) and two tendons (peroneus brevis and peroneus tertius).

Iselin disease is defined as an overuse injury caused by repetitive pressure and/or traction on the growth center at the base of the fifth metatarsal. It is subsequent to the tension produced by the peroneus brevis muscle tendon and is especially found in young athletic males with tight calf muscles. It is often misdiagnosed as a fracture.

The normal apophysis is usually seen between ages 10 and 14. The apophyseal line runs parallel to the shaft of metatarsal along the tubercle's inferolateral margin. It does not extend proximally into the joint.

Pain is most commonly found along the foot's outer edge. It worsens with activity and improves with rest. It is usually self-limiting, but if bone maturity is reached and symptoms continue, the injury can develop into a nonunion.

The diagnosis of Iselin disease is made primarily based on the clinical presentation and physical exam. Radiographs are useful to exclude other causes of foot pain. It usually is not visible on anteroposterior or lateral radiographs, but can be seen on the oblique view. They can help in assessing for displacement of the growth center.

Differential diagnosis for fifth metatarsal diseases includes:

- *Jone's fracture*: transverse fracture at the diaphysis/metaphysis junction. It extends from the lateral aspect of the fifth metatarsal towards the articular surface between metatarsals four and five. It is generally caused by tensile stress along the metatarsal's lateral border.
- *Stress fracture of the proximal fifth metatarsal*: transverse diaphyseal pathological fracture at the proximal 1.5 cm of the shaft. It is described in Case 4.8.
- *Avulsion fracture*: when the proximal portion of the fifth metatarsal is fractured off secondary to a violent contraction of the peroneus brevis during sudden foot inversion. The fracture line appears in the transverse plane; sometimes it can be slightly oblique.
- *Os vesalium*: accessory bone found proximal to the base of the fifth metatarsal within the peroneus brevis tendon.

Treatment is aimed to reduce pain and inflammation. Depending on symptom severity, treatment may include rest from any aggravating activities; ice massage to the inflamed area; stretching of calf and peroneal muscles; custom foot orthotics to address postural abnormalities and relieve the pressure on the growth plate; and protective, stable footwear to support the foot while the area heals. In our case, this patient (who also had a subchondral cuboid fracture) remained at rest for 38 days.

Radiological Findings

Coronal fat-suppressed MR FSE T2- and PD-weighted images of the foot (Fig. 4.5) reveals edema of the apophysis of the base of the fifth metatarsal (open arrow).

The axial T1 spin eco-weighted image (Fig. 4.6) shows the apophysis (open arrow) and, incidentally, a small subchondral cuboid fracture (arrowhead). The acute cuboid edema and the traction injury at the fifth metatarsal's apophysis are clearly appreciated in the axial FSE T2 fat-saturated weighted images (Fig. 4.7).

A normal apophysis of another 12-year-old soccer player with fifth metatarsal pain is seen in an oblique plain radiograph (Fig. 4.8).

Case 4.3: Freiberg's Infraction

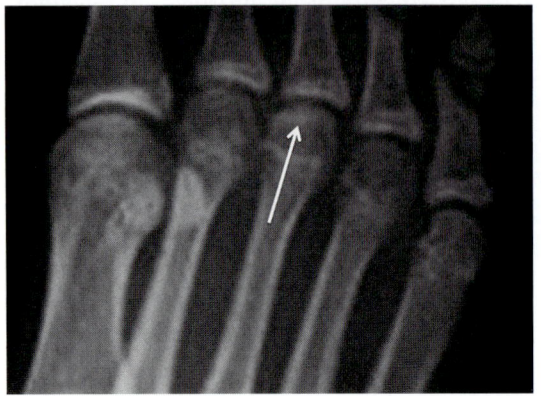

Fig. 4.9

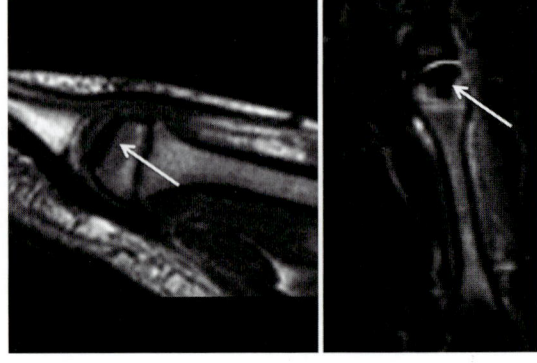

Fig. 4.10

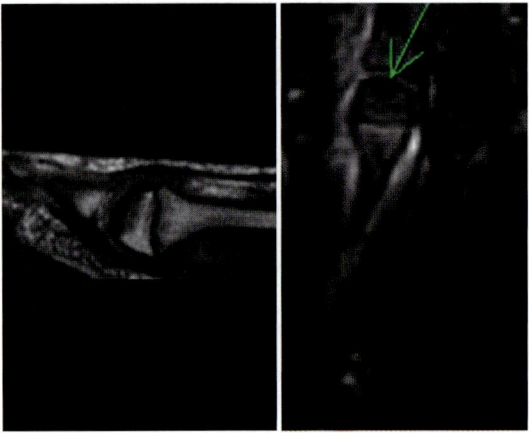

Fig. 4.11

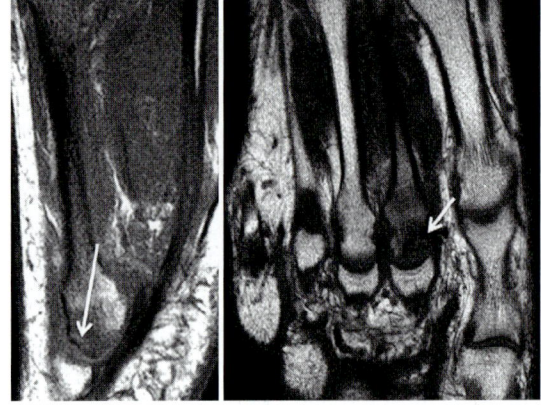

Fig. 4.12

A 16-year-old female rhythmic gymnast suffered from anterior right foot pain during training.

Comments

Freiberg's infraction is an osteochondrosis (intraarticular) that is preferentially located at the epiphyseal nucleus of the head of the second metatarsal, but can be found, less frequently, at the third metatarsal. The disease progression and imaging are the same as usual for osteochondrosis.

Several synonyms have been used to described Freiberg's infraction including: Freiberg's infarction, osteochondrosis of the second metatarsal head, eggshell fracture, Koehler second disease, Panner disease of the metatarsal, osteochondritis deformans metatarso-juvenilis, malacopathia, subchondral bone fatigue fracture of the second metatarsal head, and dorsal fatigue stress injury of the second metatarsal head.

Freiberg's infraction is a relatively common osteochondrosis of the second metatarsal head. It appears to affect young women who are active in sports. Its etiology is thought to be traumatic in nature causing a painful alteration, subchondral disruption, and collapse of the articular cartilage. "Infraction" is sometimes called Freiberg's "infarction." Infarction would suggest a vascular event leading to osteonecrosis. It has been suggested that avascular necrosis from injury will lead to the growth plate or epiphyseal injury in young, growing bone. This may also explain why the incidence is higher in young women and girls. The location and radiographic appearance of metatarsal head subchondral fractures are similar to those seen in Freiberg's infraction. The term infraction refers to an incomplete fracture of bone without displacement of fragments.

Although Freiberg's infraction affects adolescents (12–18 years) and metatarsal head subchondral fractures are seen in adults, both entities likely share a cause that combines mechanical stress, subchondral fracture, vascular injury, and subsequent osteonecrosis. Therefore, it is possible that Freiberg's infraction and metatarsal head subchondral fractures occurring in adults have the same pathogenesis.

Diagnosis is often confirmed by simple radiographs which show varying stages of metatarsal head injury and articular depression. MRI aids in the diagnosis of Freiberg's infraction before joint changes occur on radiograph. This may be particularly useful in the early stage of the disorder when joint pain is present without observed changes to the joint surface, and MRI can detect edema. There might be incidental detection of asymptomatic osteochondrosis such as the present case on the contralateral foot.

Radiological Findings

Plain radiograph (Fig. 4.9) shows slight sclerosis within the third metatarsal head (arrow) of the right foot. MRI shows significant edema through the third metatarsal with low signal on sagittal T1 and STIR coronal view (Fig. 4.10) within the head of the metatarsal due to necrosis (arrows). Figure 4.11 shows an asymptomatic osteochondrosis on the second metatarsal of the left foot (arrow).

Figure 4.12 depicts a metatarsal head subchondral fracture of a 63-year-old female. Sagittal and coronal T1-weighted images show metatarsal head flattening (long arrow) involving dorsal surface with subchondral sclerosis (short arrow).

Case 4.4: Physeal Widening of the Distal Femur and Proximal Tibia

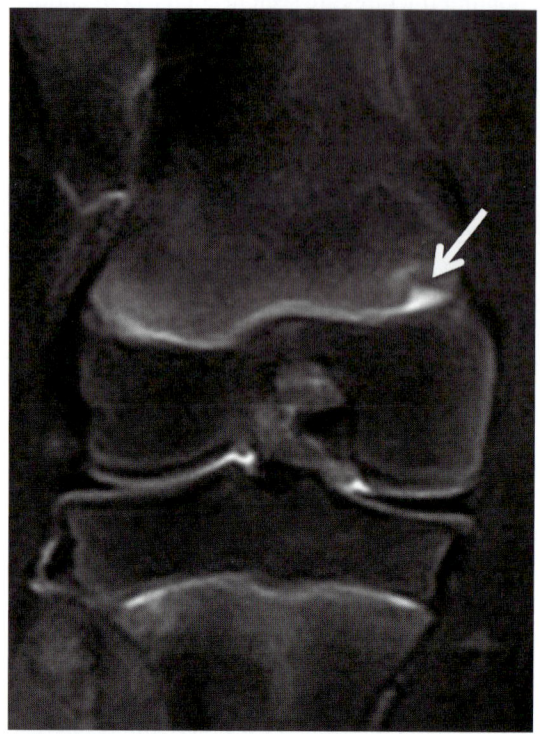

Fig. 4.13

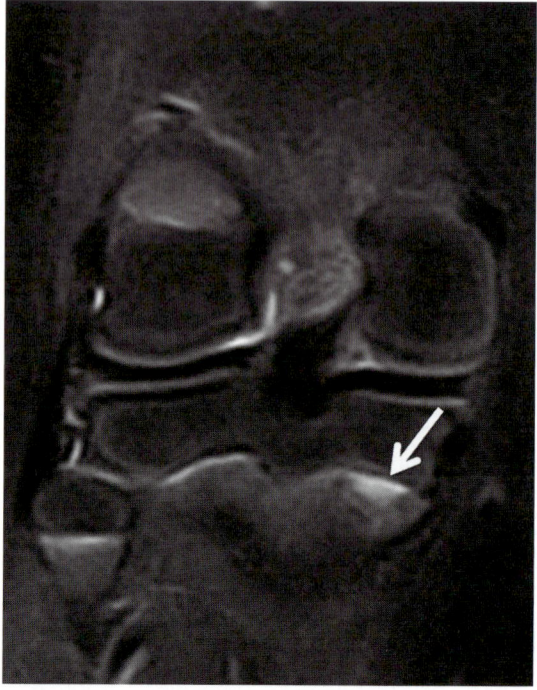

Fig. 4.14

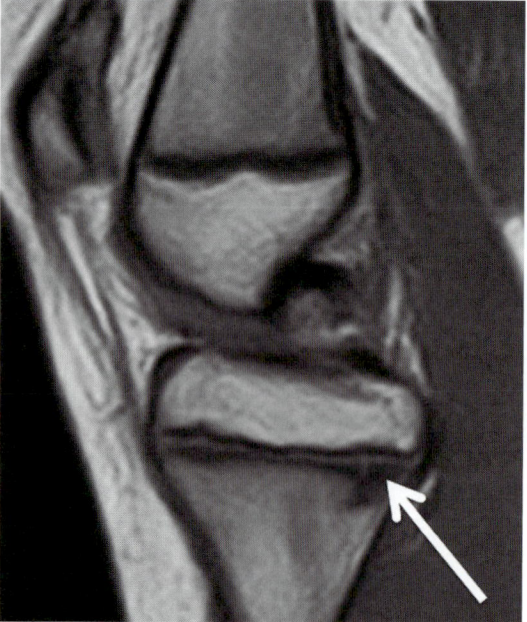

Fig. 4.15

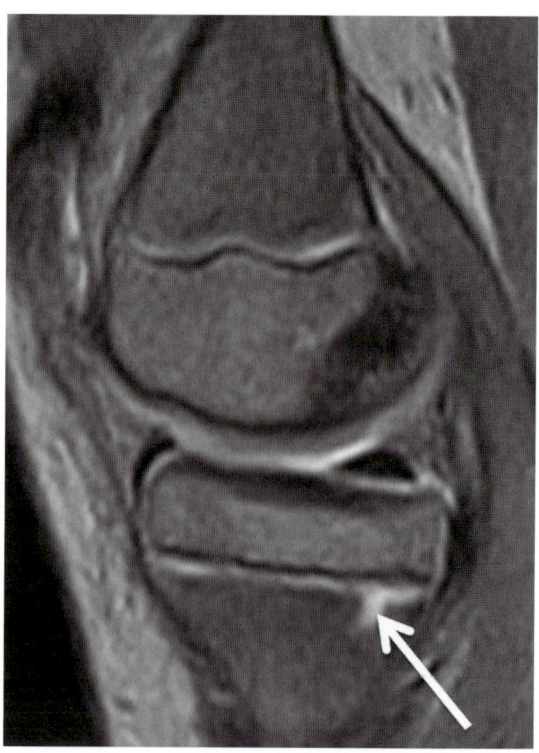

Fig. 4.16

A 13-year-old male tennis player complains of knee pain during the last 3 weeks without any related traumatic event.

Comments

Physeal widening can be observed on MRI of children as the result of a variety of metaphyseal insults. The widening may be broad or more focal. These areas of physeal widening differ from Salter-Harris type 1 injuries in that no discrete fracture is identified through the cartilage, the widening can be quite focal, and neither epiphyseal nor apophyseal displacement is seen.

Salter-Harris fractures are often the result of an acute insult or injury in children, whereas broad physeal widening is suggestive of chronic stress. This form of repetitive microtrauma results in the equivalent of a stress injury disrupting the microvascular blood supply to the physis, thereby interrupting normal endochondral bone formation. The term "epiphysiolysis" has been used in this respect, especially in the humerus, but it is potentially misleading since it could imply separation of the epiphysis from the proximal shaft or a fracture through the epiphysis itself, neither of which is expected here.

This condition is associated with knee pain but not related to an acute traumatic event, although it is referred with an intense sport activity. Usually these children are high-intensity, competitive elite, or subelite athletes who participate in sports, beyond the recreational level. Extension of physeal signal intensity into the adjacent metaphysis of bones has been described on MRI in both symptomatic and asymptomatic children. The newly formed metaphyseal bone immediately adjacent to the physis is relatively fragile and has poor resistance to compressive forces, such as those from the chronic stress of competitive sports activity. The radiologist may be the first to recognize the physeal widening seen on imaging and to suggest that this finding is a possible form of stress injury in competitive, skeletally immature athletes. MRI in children with overuse pain may be performed to confirm physeal widening detected on radiography and to exclude other injuries that may cause prolonged joint pain.

Treatment is conservative which consists of relative rest with an average period of 3 months.

Radiological Findings

Coronal STIR MR imaging (Figs. 4.13 and 4.14) shows physeal widening of medial aspect of the distal femoral and proximal tibial physis (arrows).

Sagittal T1 (Fig. 4.15) and GRE T2 (Fig. 4.16) shows the physeal widening of the posterior tibia (arrows) with similar high signal to that of rest of the physis (Fig. 4.16).

Case 4.5: Premature Physeal Arrest of the Distal Tibia

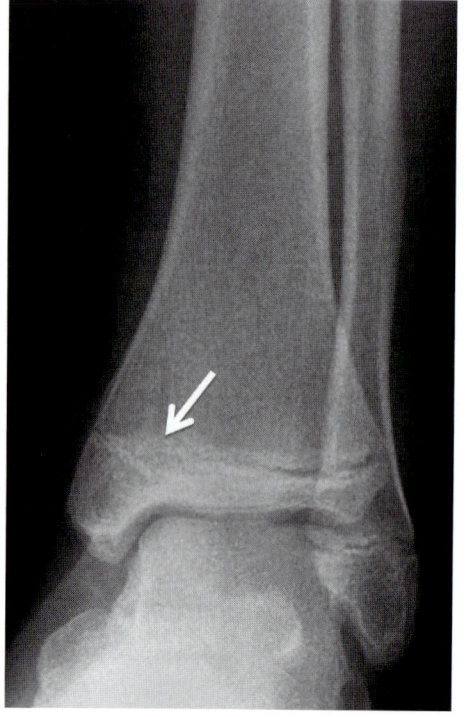

Fig. 4.17

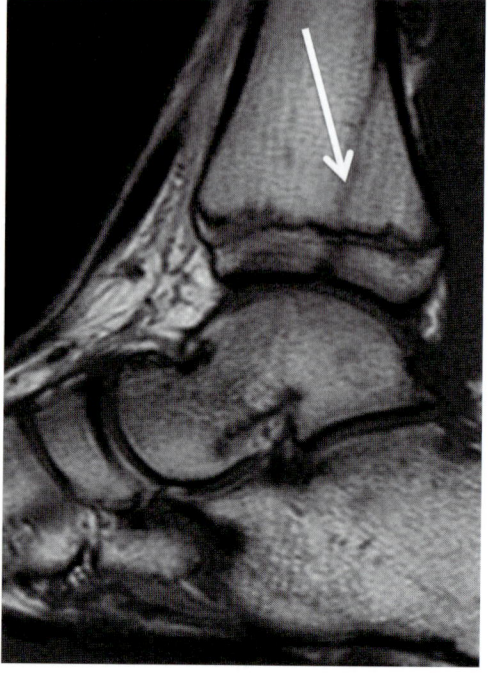

Fig. 4.18

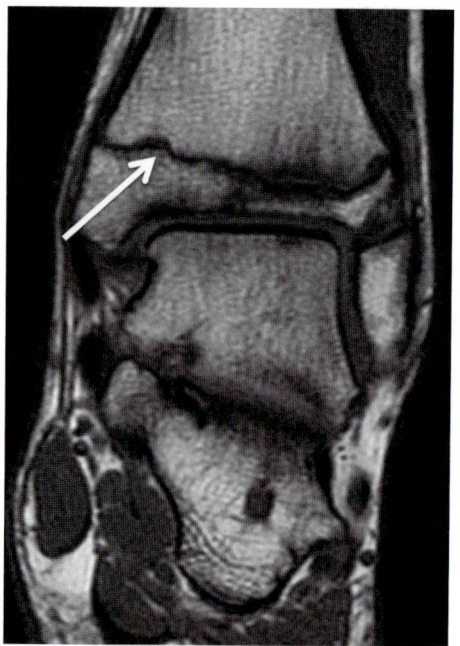

Fig. 4.19

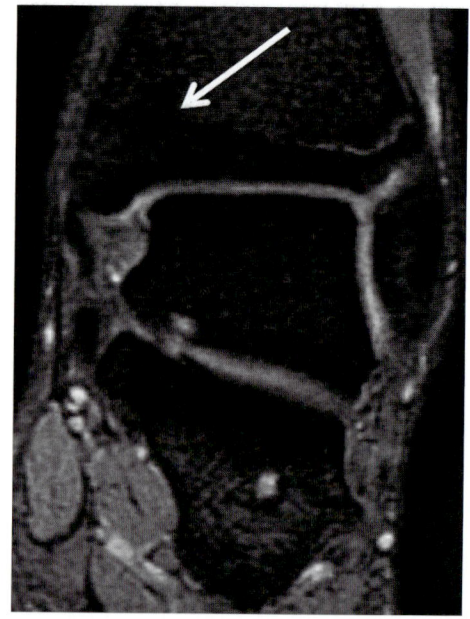

Fig. 4.20

A 14-year-old male soccer player suffered a fracture of the tibia, type Salter-Harris IV. An MRI was requested for follow-up.

Comments

Disturbance of skeletal growth occurs most frequently after trauma but may also result from other insults such as infection, ischemia, tumoral invasion, and radiation. Physeal injuries lead to premature growth arrest due to the formation of an osseous connection or bone bridge, between the epiphysis and metaphysis across the physis. If the bridge is large and centrally located in the physis, growth is slowed or stopped and limb shortening results. If the bridge is small but peripheral, growth is tethered and angular deformity develops.

Fracture across the physis, especially if vertical as the present case of Salter-Harris type 4, permits transphyseal vascular communication between the epiphysis and metaphysis. Osteoprogenitor cells accompany the vessels and deposit bone leading to a bridge across the physis. The most frequent site of posttraumatic bridge formation is the distal tibia, where a longitudinal fracture might extend from the epiphysis to the metaphysis perpendicular to the plane of the physis.

The goal of imaging patients with growth disturbance is accurate demonstration of the physeal cartilaginous pathology and depiction of the size and location of bone bridges relative to the remainder of the physis to guide surgical management. Radiography, tomography, scintigraphy, and CT have been used to evaluate patients with growth arrest. Unfortunately, all of these techniques are limited in their ability to define the relationship of the bone bridge to the cartilaginous physis.

MR imaging has become the modality of choice to evaluate physeal abnormalities. Normal physiologic closure of this physis begins at an anteromedial undulation called Kump's bump, which can be seen radiographically and with MR imaging. This is also the most common location for posttraumatic premature physeal closure of the distal tibia. The physeal bone bridges appear as low-signal-intensity areas within the otherwise high-signal-intensity physis or as an area of physeal narrowing. Bridging usually occurs at the undulations where physiologic closure begins.

The early detection of the physeal arrest in this patient led to perform operative treatment with epiphyseodesis. The patient had complete recovery and still is active in playing soccer.

Radiological Findings

Plain film (Fig. 4.17) shows sclerosis and premature fusion of medial distal tibial physis (*arrow*) with angular deformity. Growth recovery line and physis converge at bridge (arrow).

Sagittal T1-weighted image (Fig. 4.18) shows the consolidated longitudinal fracture (arrow)

Coronal T1-weighted image (Fig. 4.19) demonstrates Kump's bump, which is the site of initial physiologic physeal closure and the most common location of posttraumatic premature physeal bridging (arrow)

Coronal gradient echo T2-weighted image (Fig. 4.20) shows physeal bridge as an area of physeal narrowing and diminished signal intensity (arrow)

Case 4.6: Osteochondritis Dissecans of the Knee

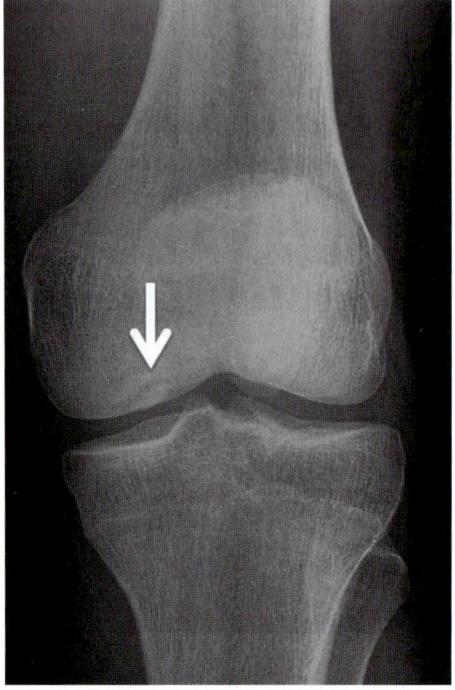

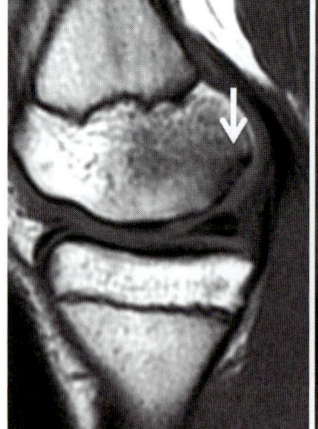

Fig. 4.22

Fig. 4.21

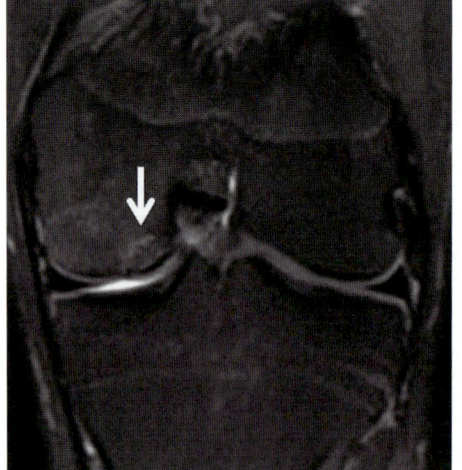

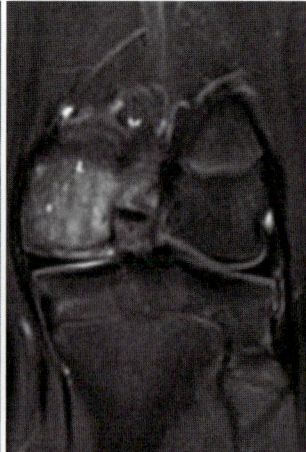

Fig. 4.23

Fig. 4.24

A 15-year-old boy sustained an injury 2 years ago. Two weeks prior to MR imaging, he developed pain on his left knee without a specific inciting event.

Comments

Osteochondritis dissecans (OCD) is an acquired condition affecting subchondral bone that manifests as a pathological spectrum including softening of the overlying articular cartilage with an intact articular surface, early articular cartilage separation, partial detachment of an articular lesion, and osteochondral separation with loose bodies. The etiology of OCD remains speculative; however, repetitive microtrauma is a common association.

OCD of the knee, the most commonly affected joint in the body, is categorized into juvenile and adult forms based on the status of the distal femoral physis. The juvenile form occurs in children 5–15 years of age with open growth plates, whereas the adult form occurs in skeletally mature patients ages 16–50 years. Ultimately, the prognosis of this acquired disorder depends on the status of the growth plate because skeletally mature patients often fail conservative management and frequently require operative intervention for complete healing.

Diagnostic imaging studies, such as plain radiographs and magnetic resonance imaging, should be performed when appropriate to characterize the lesion in terms of size and location and to determine whether it is stable, unstable, or a full-thickness defect with or without loose bodies.

MRI should be performed to elucidate the size of the lesion and the status of the subchondral bone and overlying cartilage. Other important findings on MRI include the degree of bone edema, the presence of a high signal zone beneath the fragment, and the presence of loose bodies.

MRI finding on T2-weighted images of a high signal line behind the OCD fragment has been found to have a large predictive value in determining unstable lesions. A breach in the cartilage observed on T1-weighted MRI also may help predict treatment failure, particularly when observed in conjunction with a high signal line on T2-weighted images.

Unstable lesions, or knees with loose bodies, torn menisci, or any other operative intra-articular pathology, warrant initial arthroscopic evaluation and treatment. There is widespread agreement that initial nonoperative management is indicated for stable OCD lesions, as the natural history is generally favorable in a child with open physes.

Grade-I OCD could be confused with variants of ossification during normal development of the knee. Features to distinguish normal variants from OCD are location in the inferocentral posterior femoral condyles with intact overlying articular cartilage, accessory ossification centers, spiculations, residual cartilaginous model, and lack of bone marrow edema. These findings are discussed in length within a normal variant case of Chap. 5 (Case 5.4).

Radiological Findings

Anteroposterior radiograph (Fig. 4.21) and MRI (Figs. 4.22 and 4.23) show a stage 2 juvenile OCD lesion of the medial femoral condyle. The lesion is clearly demarcated from the underlying subchondral bone; however, the articular surface appears intact. There is neither high signal line on gradient echo T2-WI (Fig. 4.22) nor edema on fat-suppression T2-WI (Fig. 4.23) due to the chronic event. Figure 4.24 shows a separate case of an OCD grade-I, demonstrating a posteroinferior subchondral low signal on the sagittal T1 WI. The presence of edema within the condyle on fat-suppression T2 WI helps to distinguish the lesion from a normal variant.

Case 4.7: Fibula Stress Fracture

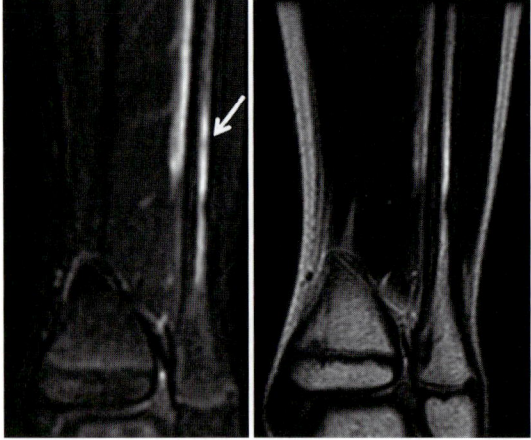

Fig. 4.25

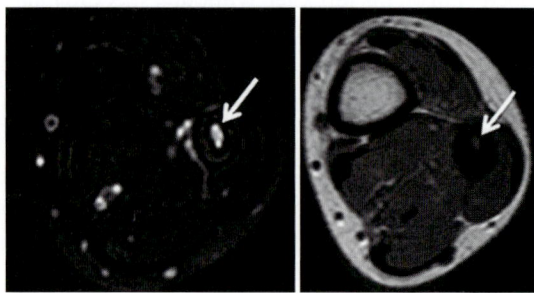

Fig. 4.26

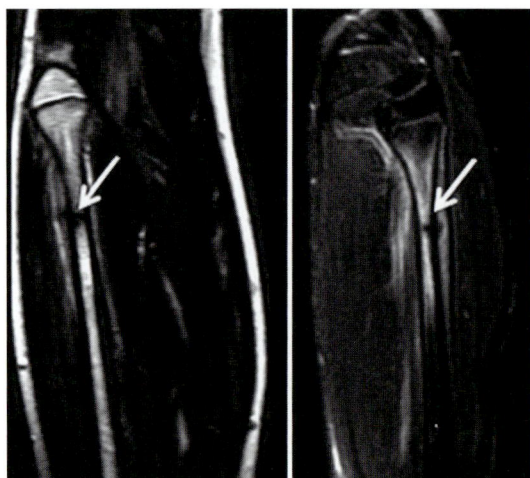

Fig. 4.27

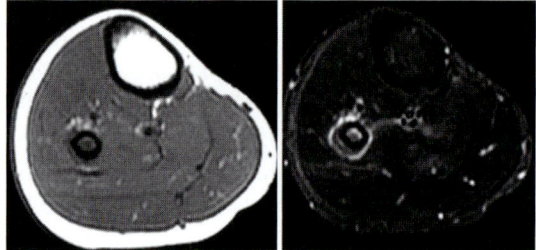

Fig. 4.28

A 7-year-old male complained from pain of the left ankle restricting the sports activity.

Comments

A stress fracture is an overuse injury. The bone is constantly attempting to remodel and repair itself, especially when extraordinary stress is applied. When enough stress is placed on the bone, it causes an imbalance between osteoclastic and osteblastic activity, and a stress fracture may appear. Muscle fatigue can also play a role in the occurrence of stress fractures. The lower limb is most commonly involved in this type of lesion, particularly at the level of the diaphysis of the tibia and fibula and especially in runners. They typically present with swelling and pain that correlates to the physical activity, but without a precise and reliable history for direct acute trauma.

Radiographs have a sensitivity of 15–35 % for detecting stress fractures on initial examinations, increasing to 30–70 % at follow-up due to more obvious bone reaction. Therefore, radiologists should not be comforted by negative radiographs and should initiate further state of the art imaging. Radiographs are however mandatory in order to show obvious fractures and to rule out other diseases, like infections or tumors, especially in children.

Stress fractures radiographically might show the following signs: in cortical bone, endosteal or periosteal callus formation without fracture line, circumferential periosteal reaction with fracture line through one cortex, and/or frank fracture. In the cancellous bone, flake-like patches of new bone formation (2–3 weeks), cloud-like area of mineralized bone, and/or focal linear area of sclerosis, perpendicular to the trabeculae.

MRI has surpassed bone scintigraphy as the imaging tool for stress fractures, showing equal sensitivity (100 %) but a higher specificity (85 %) and giving better anatomical detail and more precisely depicting the tissues involved. STIR (short tau inversion recovery), T1-weighted (T1WI) and T2-weighted images (T2WI) are used for characterization and grading. Grading is based on signs seen at MRI: (1) mild–moderate periosteal edema on STIR, no marrow changes; (2) moderate–severe periosteal edema on STIR + marrow changes on T2WI; (3) 2 + marrow changes on T1WI; and (4) fracture line visible.

Fibular fractures account for 10 % of stress fractures. Stress fractures of the fibula typically occur in the distal one-third.

Radiological Findings

Coronal STIR and T2-weighted images (Fig. 4.25) show edema on STIR (arrow) and a diffuse cortical thickening from the fibula. Axial STIR and T1-weighted images (Fig. 4.26) demonstrate also the cortical thickening and edema on T1-WI and STIR (arrows) related to a stress lesion grade 3 without fracture line.

Figure 4.27 (sagittal T2-WI and fat-suppression T2-WI) and Fig. 4.28 (axial T1-WI and fat-suppression T2-WI) show a stress fracture grade 4 of the fibula from another patient with fracture line (arrows).

Case 4.8: Proximal Diaphysis Fracture of the Fifth Metatarsal

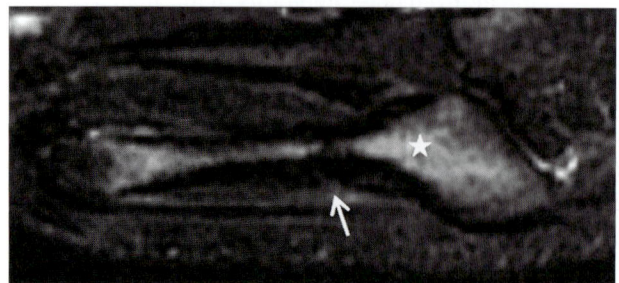

Fig. 4.29

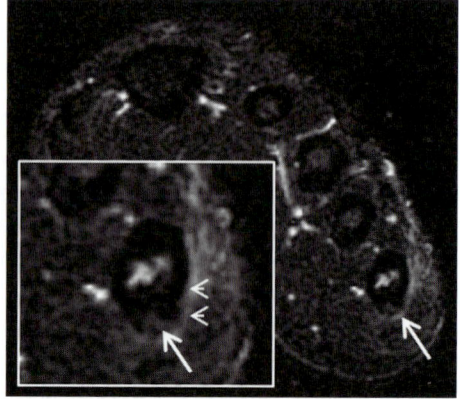

Fig. 4.30

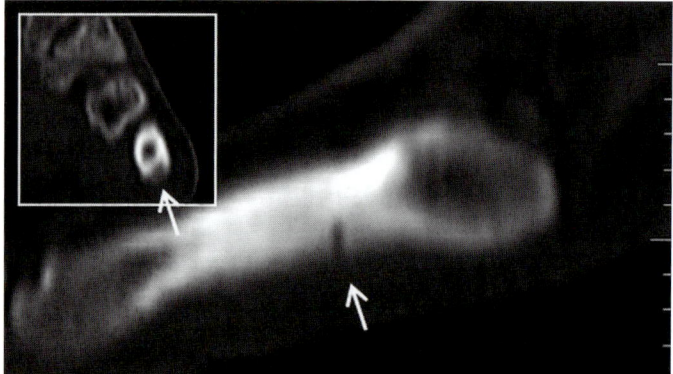

Fig. 4.31

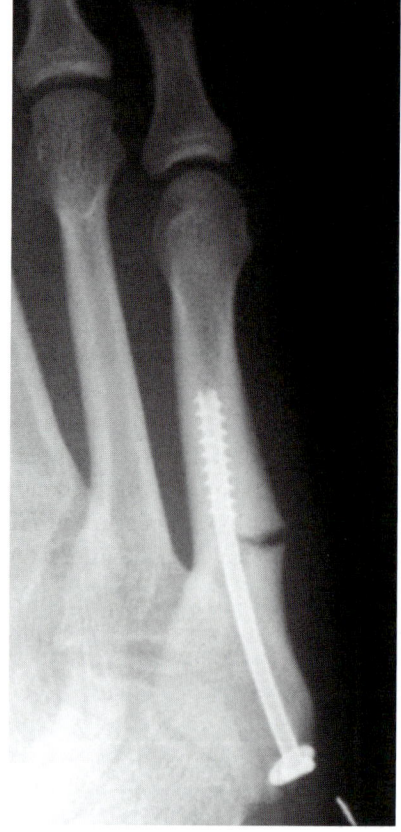

Fig. 4.32

A 17-year-old soccer player reporting foot pain during practice without previous traumatic contact

Comments

Proximal diaphysis fractures of the fifth metatarsal seen in athletes (i.e., soccer players) are frequently caused by stress. They are considered high risk with a bad outcome. Their treatment is still a challenge.

There are three separate fracture zones with different outcomes:

- Zone 1 injury: avulsion fracture at the metatarsal base. It can extend into the metatarsocuboid joint. It usually results from an indirect mechanism of injury, such as acute foot inversion.
- Zone 2 injury: transverse fracture at the proximal diaphysis – metaphyseal junction (Jones' fracture). It extends from the lateral aspect of the fifth metatarsal towards the articular surface between metatarsals four and five. It is generally caused by tensile stress along the metatarsal's lateral border.
- Zone 3 injury: *stress fracture (fatigue)* in the shaft's proximal 1.5 cm. It originates from repetitive cyclic loading. It can be associated to cavovarus foot alignment.

Zone 1 fractures have a good outcome with medical treatment (non-weight-bearing cast). Zone 2 and 3 fractures can be prone to complications. The vascular watershed area within the proximal diaphysis may be the reason for high rates of nonunion, delayed union, and re-fracture in this region.

MRI can be useful as the first step in diagnosis when the bone stress reaction is seen as bone marrow edema without fracture. The complete or incomplete cortical fracture can be appreciated in X-ray, CT, and MRI.

Treatment of proximal diaphysis fractures of the fifth metatarsal is still a challenge. Conservative treatment is the first step in incomplete fractures (such as the one seen in our soccer player). Operative fixation (percutaneous bicortical or intramedullary) with optional bone grafting shortens recovery time with decreased rates of nonunion, delayed union, and re-fracture. For these reasons and in order to allow faster return to sporting activity, fixation is performed in athletes even with non-displaced fractures.

These fractures used to take long periods to recover. Our player was out of action for 2 weeks and returned to play asymptomatic until pain recurred during practice 2 months later. An incomplete inferior cortical fracture was seen at this time. He rested again and was able to play for 11 days without pain until he developed a near complete fracture.

Radiological Findings

Fifth metatarsal bone marrow edema (asterisk) and cortical reabsorption of the thickened inferior cortex (thick arrows) are seen in the sagittal (Fig. 4.29) and coronal (Fig. 4.30) FSE T2 fat-saturated weighted images. Periosteal edema is seen surrounding the cortex (thin arrows).

An incomplete cortical fracture (arrow) is seen in the sagittal reconstruction and axial plane CT (Fig. 4.31) 2 months later. After playing again with no pain, he developed a near complete fracture (Fig. 4.32) 2 weeks later. This time, unlike at the beginning of the process, internal fixation was required.

Case 4.9: Early Lumbar Spondylolysis

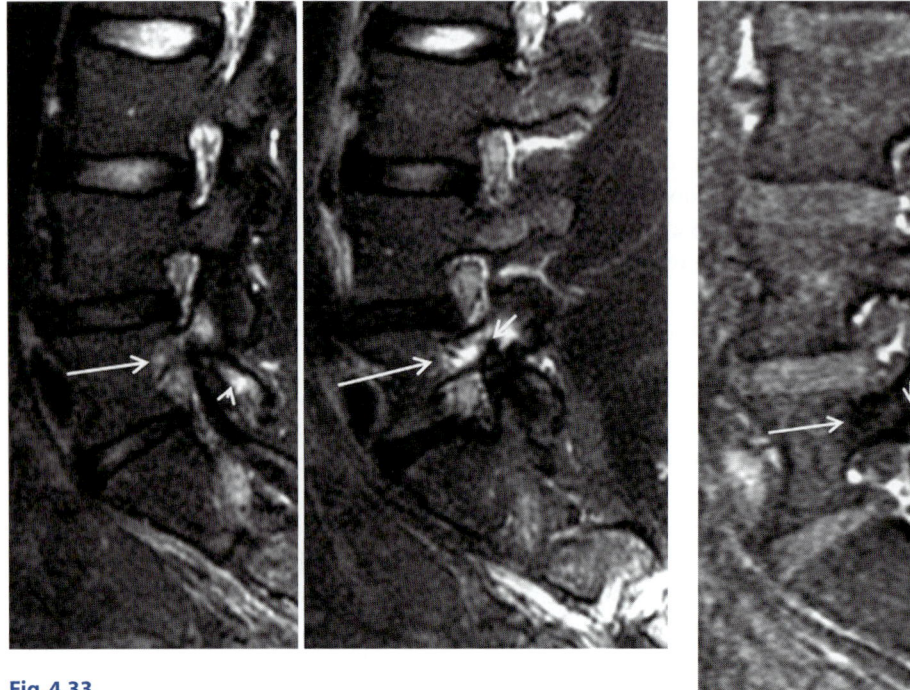

Fig. 4.33

Fig. 4.34

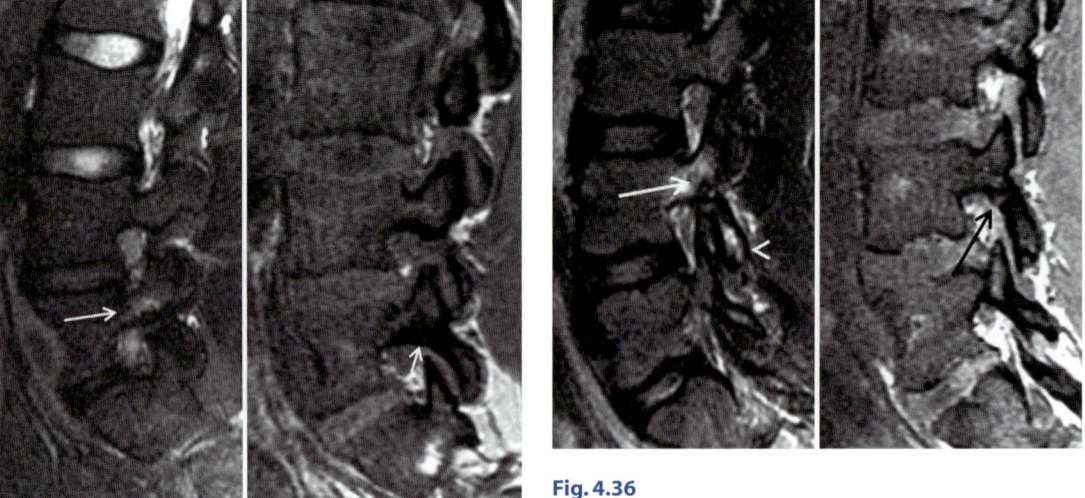

Fig. 4.36

Fig. 4.35

A 17-year-old soccer play, complaining of low back pain for 2 weeks. The unipodal spinal hyperextension test was positive. Nothing abnormal was evident in plain radiographs.

Comments

Lumbar spondylolysis is a very common cause of low back pain in young athletes (up to 47 %). It is caused by a pars interarticularis defect with a high incidence (68 % by some authors) in those practicing sports that combine repetitive flexion, extension, and rotation of the lumbar spine (tennis, baseball, soccer, gymnastics, weight lifting, rowing, etc.). Although multiple factors may be involved in its genesis, when it occurs in juvenile athletes, it is currently considered a stress fracture resulting from repetitive microtrauma on a predisposed weak area.

It is commonly seen between ages 10–18. The spondylolysis is found predominantly at L5 level, since, in daily activities, it is subjected to the greatest amount of static and dynamic stress. Its incidence decreases proceeding cephalad. It is most frequently bilateral. The defect begins in the inferior cortex between the pedicle and the pars.

This type of stress fracture develops in stages. The first stage is a radiographically and CT occult stress-related injury to the pars without cortical interruption (*stage 1*). Over time and with continued insult, this can progress to an incomplete stress fracture (*stage 2*); then complete acute pars stress fracture (*stage 3*); and then, if healing and reunion do not occur, it eventually develops into a chronic inactive nonunion (*stage 4*).

MR imaging can be used as the first-line noninvasive investigation for juvenile spondylolysis. It has the potential to detect early bone marrow edema (secondary to the pars and pedicle stress) and, with the appropriate imaging sequences (FSE T2 FAT SAT or STIR and 3D SPGR sequences) to examine the inferior cortical reabsorption area or incomplete fracture. MRI can also rule out associated disk degeneration, disk herniation, or spina bifida (with 3D SPGR).

Stress reaction and incomplete fracture diagnosis is important as fracture healing may be achieved with conservative treatment alone, preventing progression to pseudoarthrosis, which, in itself, has a higher incidence of spondylolisthesis.

These fractures usually take long periods to recover. Our player used an antilordotic brace for 6 weeks and was out of action for 3 months.

Radiological Findings

Pedicle bone marrow edema (long arrow) and pars (arrowhead) are clearly seen on the left side of this L5 vertebra in these two continuous sagittal FSE T2 fat-saturated weighted images (Fig. 4.33). In this sequence, a line can be faintly seen in the inferior cortex (short arrow). The incomplete stress fracture in the inferior cortex (short arrow) is clearly defined in the 3D-spoiled gradient echo (SPGR) (Fig. 4.34). An MRI 3 months later (Fig. 4.35) shows healing with inferior cortical sclerosis without fracture (short arrow) and no pedicle edema (long arrow).

A grade 2 fracture in another 15-year-old soccer player (Fig. 4.36) shows L4 pars and pedicle edema on the right side with an incomplete inferior fracture clearly defined in the 3D SPGR image (black arrow).

Case 4.10: Bilateral Pedicular Stress Fracture

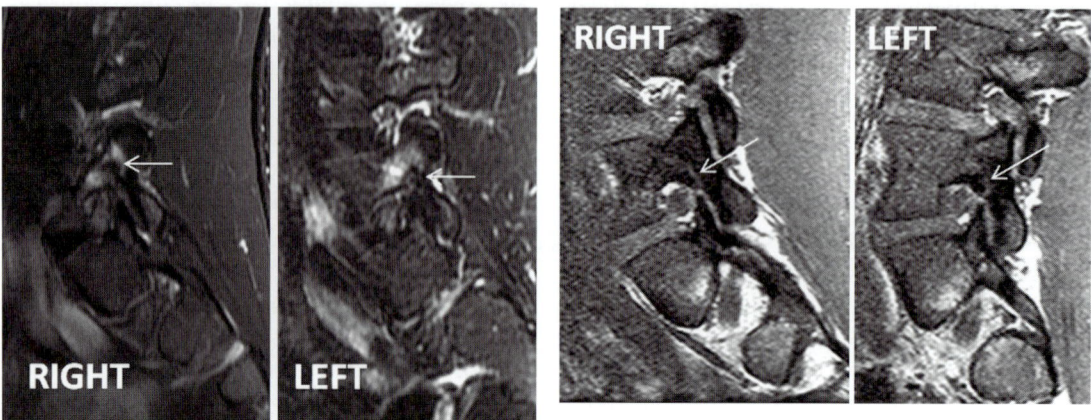

Fig. 4.37

Fig. 4.38

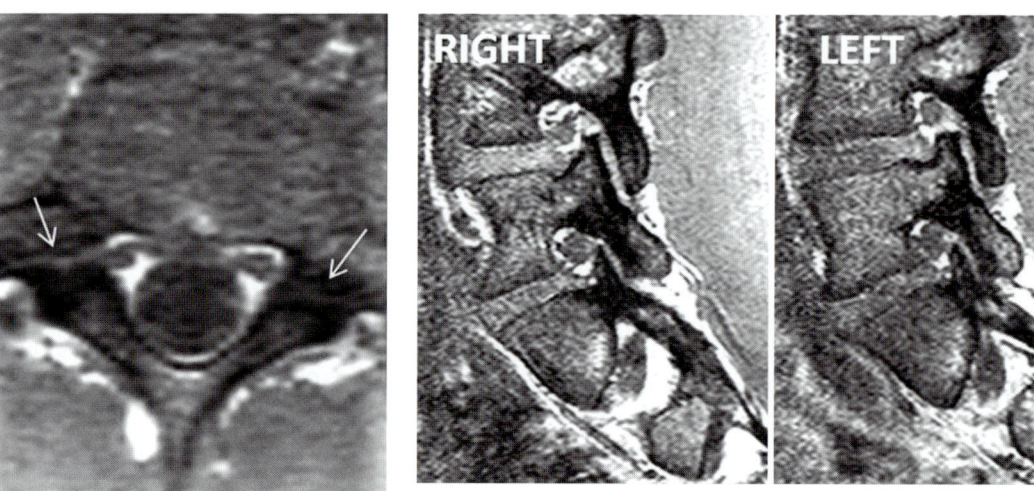

Fig. 4.39

Fig. 4.40

A 17-year-old semiprofessional soccer player complained of low back pain for 3 weeks. The pain increased with lumbar hyperextension and rotational movements.

Comments

The prevalence of pedicular stress fractures (without trauma and/or previous surgery) has not been assessed. Bilateral pedicular fractures are noted to be less common than unilateral ones. Just like symptomatic spondylolysis, they can cause low back pain (which increases with lumbar movements) in young athletes.

Pedicular stress fractures are less common than those affecting the pars interarticularis, as the pedicle is the second most common point of maximal stress loading after the pars. It has been published as having a higher prevalence amongst unilateral spondylolysis cases.

Pedicle stress fractures imaging may be similar to that for pars interarticularis defects. The *stress reaction – initial stage* (without line fracture) is not seen in radiographs or CT. MRI is a useful technique at this early stage, as the pedicle edema is seen as a high intensity signal in the T2 fat-suppressed sequence. Since the pedicle, anatomically, adjoins the pars interarticularis, the pedicular changes may be consequence of both the pars' stress fracture or the pedicular fracture itself. The *incomplete fracture – next stage* (which involves the inferior cortex) is frequently

occult to X-ray, but can be seen in CT and also MRI. sagital thin-section 3D spoiled gradient echo sequence is a useful technique in demonstrating cortex integrity. The *completed fracture – last stage* (involves the superior cortex) can be seen in X-ray, CT, and MRI.

Early detection and correct treatment of these fractures, as in spondylolysis, is important to achieve bony union. Treatment for spondylolysis is initially conservative and aims to reduce pain and facilitate healing.

Players usually take quite long to recover from this disease (same as in spondylolysis). This player used an antilordotic brace for 6 weeks and took 9 weeks to return to competition. He is currently a professional soccer player.

Radiological Findings

The sagittal FSE T2 fat-saturated weighted images (Fig. 4.37) show high signal intensity due to edema in both L4 pedicles. The incomplete inferior cortical pedicular fractures are also faintly seen (arrows) in this sequence.

The pedicular fractures (arrows) are clearly defined in the 3D-spoiled gradient echo (SPGR) sequence, sagittal (Fig. 4.38), and axial reconstructions (Fig. 4.39).

The sagittal 3D-spoiled gradient echo (SPGR) (Fig. 4.40) sequence 4 months later shows sclerosis of the inferior cortex without fractures, in correlation with healing.

Further Reading

Books

Boos N, Aebi M (eds) (2008) Spinal disorders: fundamentals of diagnosis and treatment. Springer, Berlin/Heidelberg/New York

Campbell WC, Canale ST, Beaty JH (2008) Campbell's operative orthopaedics, 11th edn. Mosby/Elsevier, Philadelphia

Karantas A (2011) Sports injuries in children and adolescents. Springer, Berlin/Heidelberg

Martino F, Defilippi C, Caudana R (2009) Imaging of pediatric bone and joint trauma. Springer-Verlag, Italia

Stoller T, Bredella B, Branstetter B (2008) Diagnostic imaging orthopaedics, 1st edn. AMIRSYS, Salt Lake City

Websites

www.mskcases.com
www.radiologyeducation.com
www.radsource.us
www.uhrad.com
www.wheelessonline.com.

Articles

Bradley AM (2010) Sports-related injury of the pediatric spine. Radiol Clin North Am 48:1237–1248

Dunn AJ, Campbell RSD, Mayor PE, Rees D (2008) Radiological findings and healing patterns of incomplete stress fractures of the pars interarticularis. Skeletal Radiol 37:443–450

Ecklund K, Jaramillo D (2001) Imaging of growth disturbance in children. Radiol Clin North Am 39(4):823–841

Ecklund K, Jaramillo D (2002) Patterns of premature physeal arrest: MR imaging of 111 children. AJR Am J Roentgenol 178(4):967–972

Fetzer GB, Wright RW (2006) Metatarsal shaft fractures and fractures of the proximal fifth metatarsal. Clin Sports Med 25:139–150

Ganiyusufoglu AK, Onat L, Karatoprak O, Enercan M, Hamzaoglu A (2010) Diagnostic accuracy of magnetic resonance imaging versus computed tomography in stress fractures of the lumbar spine. Clin Radiol 65:902–907

Gebarski K, Hernandez RJ (2005) Stage-I osteochondritis dissecans versus normal variants of ossification in the knee in children. Pediatr Radiol 35(9):880–886

Hollenberg GM, Beattie PF, Meyers SP, Weinberg EP, Adams MJ (2002) Stress reactions of the lumbar pars interarticularis: the development of a New MRI classification system. Spine 27(2):181–186

Kerssemakers SP, Fotiadou AN, De Jonge MC, Karantanas AH, Maas M (2009) Sport injuries in the paediatric and adolescent patient: a growing problem. Pediatr Radiol 39:471–484

Kirkland WD (2010) Imaging pediatric sports injuries: lower extremity. Radiol Clin North Am 48:1213–1235

Kobayashi A, Kobayashi T, Kato K, Higuchi H, Takagishi K (2013) Diagnosis of radiographically occult lumbar spondylolysis in young athletes by magnetic resonance imaging. Am J Sports Med 41:169, Originally published online November 7, 2012

Kocher MS, Tucker R, Ganley TJ, Flynn JM (2006) Management of osteochondritis dissecans of the knee: current concepts review. Am J Sports Med 34(7):1181–1191

Laor T, Jaramillo D (2009) MR imaging insights into skeletal maturation: what is normal? Radiology 250(1):28–38

Laor T, Wall EJ, Vu LP (2006) Physeal widening in the knee due to stress injury in child athletes. AJR Am J Roentgenol 186(5):1260–1264

Leone A, Cianfoni A, Cerase A, Magarelli N, Bonomo L (2011) Lumbar spondylolysis: a review. Skeletal Radiol 40:683–700

Liong SY, Whitehouse RW (2012) Lower extremity and pelvic stress fractures in athletes. Br J Radiol 85(1016):1148–1156

Mahajan V, Chung HW, Suh JS (2011) Fractures of the proximal fifth metatarsal: percutaneous bicortical fixation. Clin Orthop Surg 3:140–146

Murthy NS (2012) Imaging of stress fractures of the spine. Radiol Clin North Am 50:799–821

Parvataneni HK, Nicholas SJ, McCance SE (2004) Bilateral pedicle stress fractures in a female athlete: case report and review of the literature. Spine 29(2):E19–E21

Royer M, Thomas T, Cesini J, Legrand E (2012) Stress fractures in 2011: practical approach. Joint Bone Spine 79(Suppl 2):S86–S90

Sairyo K, Katoh S, Takata Y, Terai T, Yasui N, Goel VK, Masuda A, Vadapalli S, Biyani A, Ebraheim N (2006) MRI signal changes of the pedicle as an indicator for early diagnosis of spondylolysis in children and adolescents: a clinical and biomechanical study. Spine 31(2):206–211

Sakai T, Sairyo K, Mima S, Yasui N (2010) Significance of magnetic resonance imaging signal change in the pedicle in the management of pediatric lumbar spondylolysis. Spine 35(14):E641–E645

Soprano JV, Fuchs SM (2007) Common overuse injuries in the pediatric and adolescent athlete. Clin Pediatr Emerg Med 8:7–14

Talusan PG, Diaz-Collado PJ, Reach JS Jr (2014) Freiberg's Infraction: diagnosis and treatment. Foot Ankle Spec 7(1):52–56

Torriani M, Thomas BJ, Bredella MA, Ouellette H (2008) MRI of metatarsal head subchondral fractures in patients with forefoot pain. AJR Am J Roentgenol 190(3):570–575

Miscellanea

5

Joan C. Vilanova, Sandra Baleato, and Marc-André Weber

Contents

J.C. Vilanova (✉)
Department of Radiology,
Clínica Girona-Hospital Sta. Caterina,
University of Girona, Girona, Spain
e-mail: kvilanova@comg.cat

S. Baleato
Department of Radiology,
Hospital Clínico Universitario de Santiago de
Compostela (CHUS), Santiago de Compostela
(A Coruña) 15706, Spain

M.-A. Weber
Section of Musculoskeletal Radiology,
University Hospital Heidelberg,
Heidelberg D-69118, Germany

R.M. Rodrigo et al., *Sports Injuries in Children and Adolescents*,
DOI 10.1007/978-3-642-54746-1_5, © Springer-Verlag Berlin Heidelberg 2014

Case 5.1: Femur Osteomyelitis

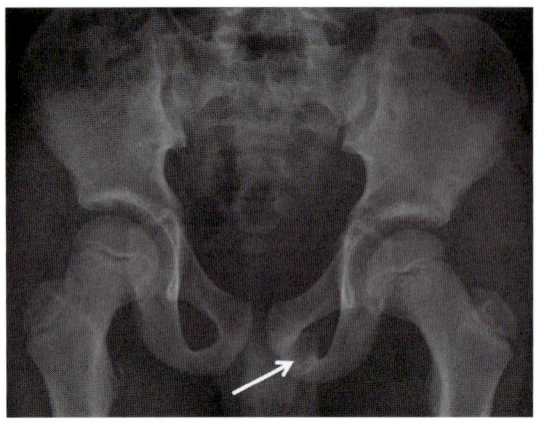

Fig. 5.1

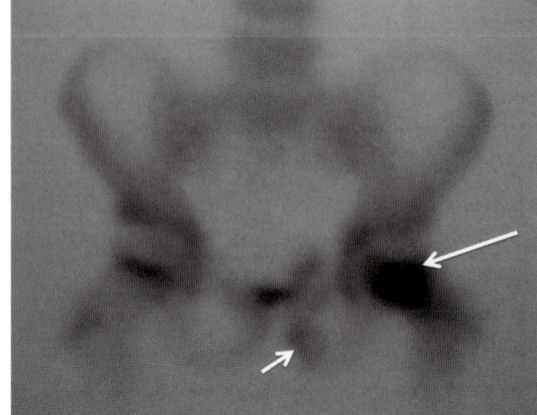

Fig. 5.2

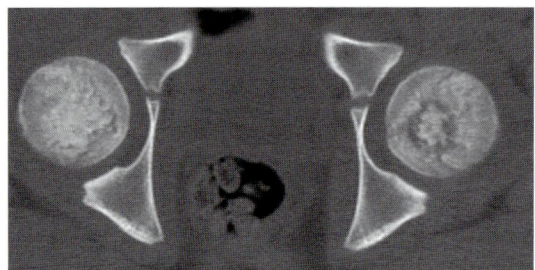

Fig. 5.3

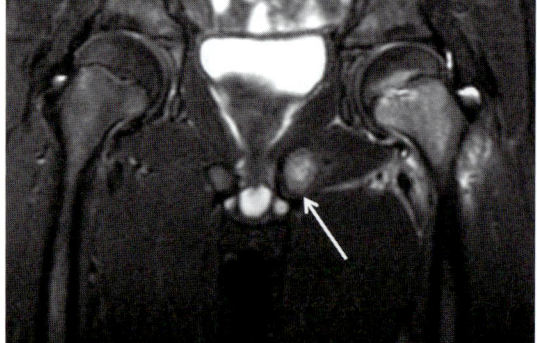

Fig. 5.4

A 9-year-old child complaining of left hip pain (restricting his soccer activities) for 3 weeks. Four weeks previously, he had suffered an abdominal superficial injury requiring subcutaneous sutures. At admission, the patient presented with intermittent fever. He had an abnormal gait and was reluctant to weight bear. A plain pelvic radiograph in the emergency room was suggestive of a left ischial bone tumor. CT, bone scintigraphy, and MRI examinations were requested.

Comments

Acute hematogenous osteomyelitis usually occurs during skeletal growth while the physis is open. Early detection is essential to start appropriate therapy before bone devitalization.

Plain x-ray manifestations may not be demonstrable for at least 10 days after onset of symptoms. The infection's evolution can show soft-tissue swelling with adjacent muscle plane obliteration, subperiosteal calcification, and bony trabecular resorption.

Bone scintigraphy is a highly sensitive procedure for diagnosing osteomyelitis. It gives a sensitive indication of altered osteoblastic activity; however, local disturbances in vascular perfusion, clearance rate, permeability, and chemical binding also affect imaging.

CT should be used as a third-line technique for visualizing bony destruction/sequestration and gas in the bone. MRI is a highly sensitive technique as a disease indicator since pathologic findings appear much earlier. The diagnosis of osteomyelitis on MRI is given by physeal bone marrow abnormalities. Active osteomyelitis appears as a low signal on T1-weighted images and a high signal on T2-weighted images, fat suppression, or STIR sequences. MR imaging is unique in being able to detect the presence of osteomyelitis and also in determining its extent.

Understanding each technique's limitations is important in order to avoid delays in the diagnosis and management of osteomyelitis and to prevent possible complications.

The differential diagnosis of pelvic osteomyelitis in children should include septic arthritis, Legg-Calve-Perthes disease, toxic synovitis, and, less commonly, collagen vascular diseases, neoplasms involving bone, or retroperitoneal abscess.

Radiological Findings

Plain pelvic radiography (Fig. 5.1) does not reveal pathologic findings suggestive of bone infection in the left femur. Incidentally a left swollen ischiopubic synchondrosis (arrow) was noted, which was initially thought to be responsible for the patient's symptoms. A bone scintigraphy scan (Fig. 5.2) shows increased uptake within the left femoral head (large arrow) and slight uptake on the left ischiopubic synchondrosis (short arrow).

CT imaging (Fig. 5.3) shows a round annular area in the left femoral head corresponding to the focal site of infection.

Coronal STIR MR imaging (Fig. 5.4) reveals femoral bone marrow high-intensity signal especially within the physis, with edema on the surrounding soft tissues. Note the ischiopubic synchondrosis hypertrophy (arrow).

Case 5.2: Adventitial Cystic Disease of the Radial Artery

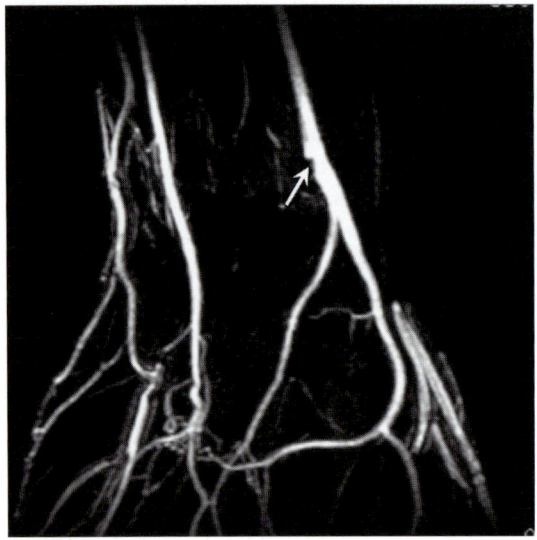

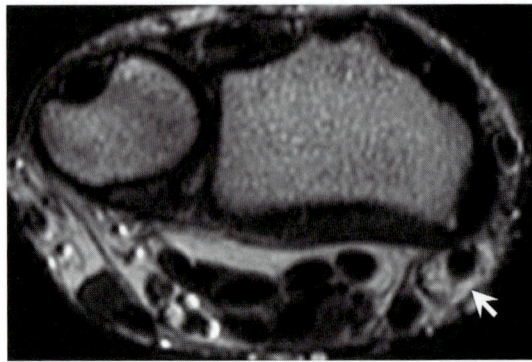

Fig. 5.6

Fig. 5.5

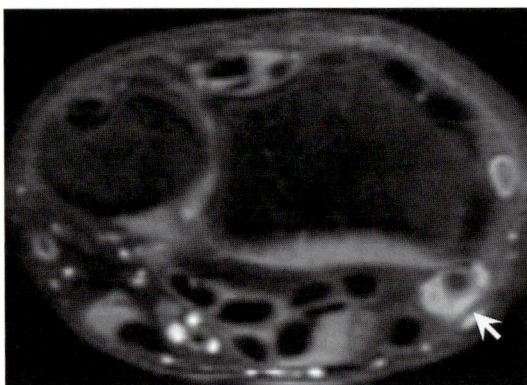

Fig. 5.7

A 17-year-old hockey player presented with recurrent pain in anatomical snuffbox after trauma 6 months ago.

Comments

Arterial adventitial cystic disease is an uncommon type of non-atherosclerotic peripheral vessel disease of unknown etiology. Several theories about their pathogenesis have been proposed such as repetitive trauma, embryological origin, direct communication with the herniated synovial structures of the adjacent joint and connective tissue disease. It affects most commonly the popliteal artery (85 % of cases), typically in young to middle-aged men without significant vascular risk factors, with a male-to-female ratio of 15:1. However, involvement of other arteries like axillary, brachial, radial, ulnar, external iliac, and common femoral has also been reported. Rarely, it can also affect the veins.

Clinically this condition results in intermittent claudication due to peripheral vascular insufficiency caused by compression of the arterial lumen by a cystic collection of mucinous material in the adventitial layer of the artery.

Magnetic resonance imaging (MRI) with magnetic resonance angiography (MRA) is very helpful in the diagnosis, as it provides excellent anatomical detail with cysts appearing as hyperintense structure on T2WI images, and luminal compromise can also be assessed.

It is an important treatable cause of vascular disease with multiple therapeutic options, which include restore arterial flow, resection of the affected artery and interposition grafting, percutaneous aspiration of cystic contents under ultrasound, or CT guidance and resectional adventitial cystotomy.

Radiological Findings

Post-contrast coronal MIP (maximal intensity projection) image from upper extremity contrast-enhanced MR angiography (Fig. 5.5) demonstrates focal narrowing of the radial artery (long arrow). The remaining vasculature is normal.

Axial T2-weighted turbo spin-echo images without (Fig. 5.6) and with fat suppression (Fig. 5.7) demonstrate a well-defined, homogeneously hyperintense cystic lesion (short arrow) corresponding to mucinous material in the adventitia layer surrounding and compressing the lumen of the radial artery.

Case 5 3: Transient Lateral Patellar Dislocation

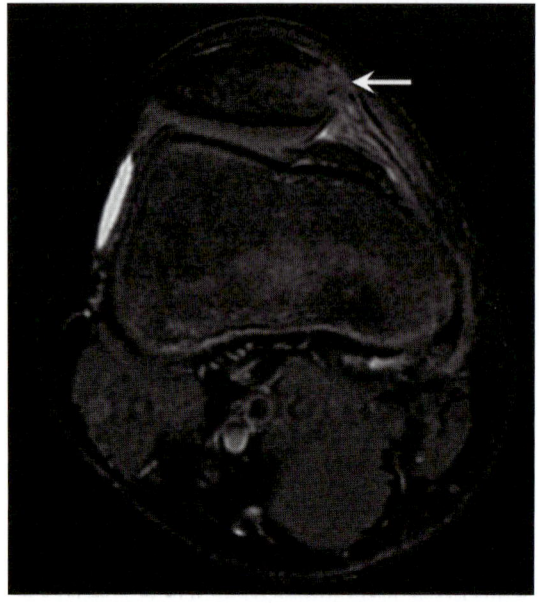

Fig. 5.8

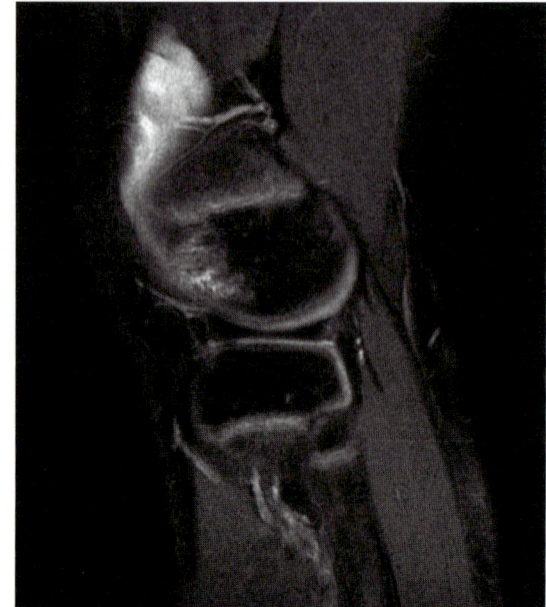

Fig. 5.9

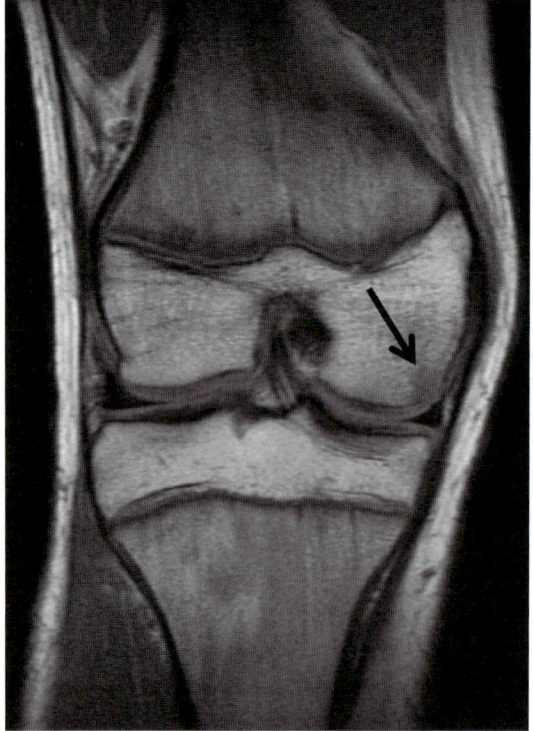

Fig. 5.10

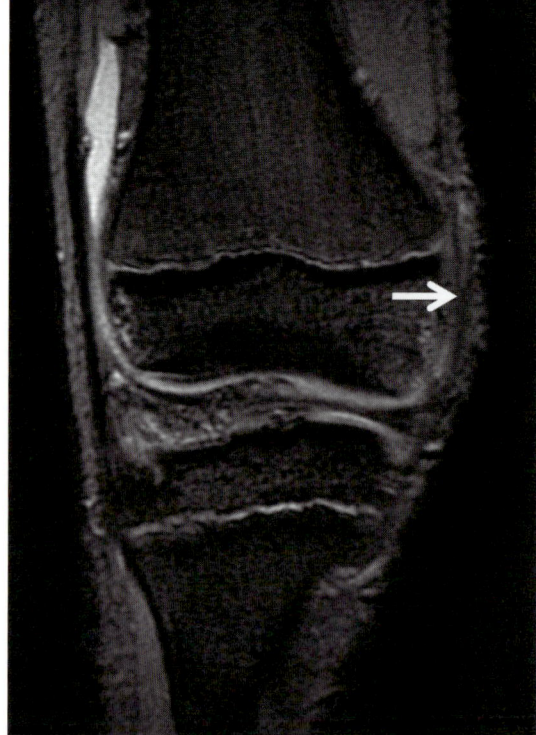

Fig. 5.11

A 13-year-old soccer player suffered a painful partial patellar dislocation while running backwards and twisting to kick the ball. The patellar subluxation reduced spontaneously. On examination, there was no ACL (anterior cruciate ligament) instability, although knee pain was persistent after the traumatic event.

Comments

Acute lateral patellar dislocation (LPD) occurs often in children during sporting activities and is commonly transient with spontaneous reduction. It accounts for approximately 9–16 % of acute knee trauma in young athletes presenting with hemarthrosis. The mechanism of injury usually involves a twisting motion: fixed foot and internal rotation on a flexed knee with valgus stress. Spontaneous relocations occur in the majority of patients. Between 50 and 75 % of diagnosis go unsuspected after clinical exam and initial plain radiology evaluation. Differentiation from other knee injuries is often difficult as extensive tenderness, hemarthrosis, and pain are often present.

Radiographs may show hemarthrosis, and a minority of patients will have a patellar chip fracture. Concomitant injuries, including medial patellofemoral ligament injuries, are common, occurring in up to 90 % of patients.

Magnetic resonance (MR) imaging findings may include typical contusion patterns in the patellar inferomedial pole and the anterolateral aspect of the femur's nonarticular portion (kissing sign) with injury to the medial patellar soft-tissue restraints. Up to one third of patients will also show concomitant injury to the major knee ligaments or menisci. These are frequently associated with osteochondral fractures, which may be an indication for surgery.

Trauma alone rarely causes patellar dislocations in patients without predisposing anatomical factors for patellar instability, such as trochlear dysplasia, dominant lateral patellar facet, high riding patella and tibial tuberosity lateralization. Trochlear dysplasia is found in up to 85 % of patients with LPD.

Nonsurgical management is generally recommended for first-time dislocations, with brace immobilization in extension for 3–6 weeks. Following initial conservative management, recurrent instability occurs in 15–50 % cases. Chronic instability and recurrent patellofemoral dislocations may cause cartilage damage with bone soft-tissue restraint abnormalities and eventual arthritic changes. Surgery may be indicated when associated injuries or abnormal patellofemoral relationships are identified.

Radiological Findings

Axial (Fig. 5.8) and sagittal (Fig. 5.9) proton density-weighted images with fat suppression reveal focal bone marrow edema involving the patellar medial aspect (arrow) and the lateral femoral condyle's lateral aspect. A medial patellar retinaculum high signal is visible without tearing. Note the trochlear dysplasia and the minimal joint effusion. Coronal T1- (Fig. 5.10) and coronal T2-GE-weighted (Fig. 5.11) MRI demonstrate focal bone marrow edema involving the medial femoral condyle with a hyperintense signal along the superficial aspect of the medial collateral ligament (MCL) (sprain grade I).

Case 5.4: Normal Knee Ossification Variants

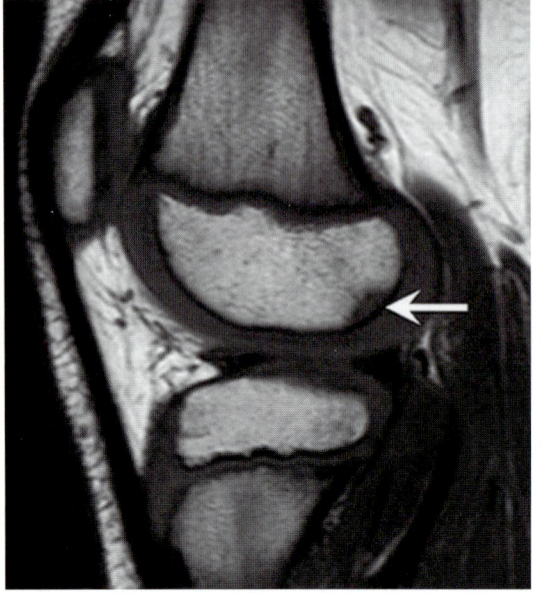

Fig. 5.12

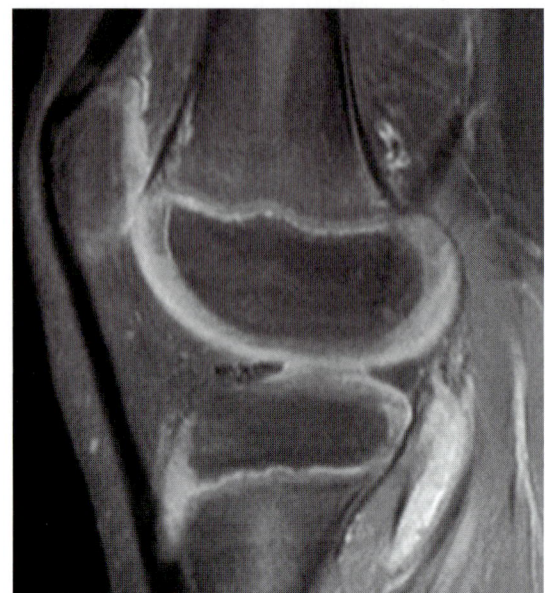

Fig. 5.13

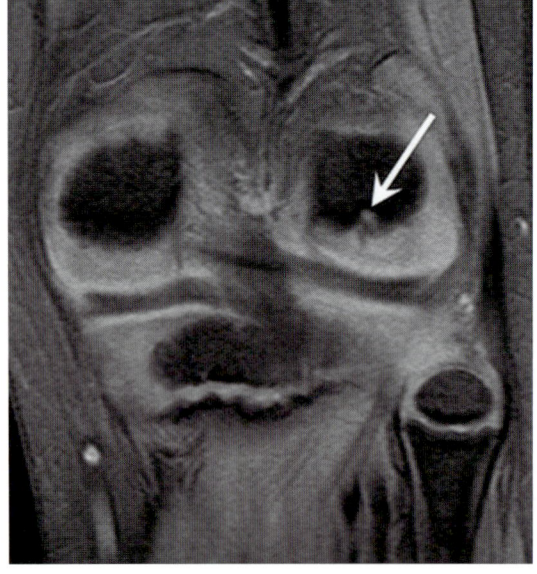

Fig. 5.14

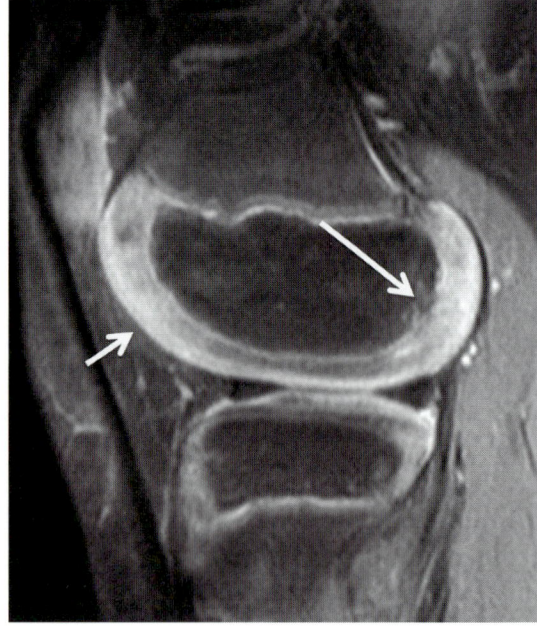

Fig. 5.15

A 7-year-old boy injured himself (internal varus mechanism) during a soccer match. He presented with bilateral knee pain (occasionally locking and more pronounced on the right) with questionable meniscal positive test. Two days later, he was asymptomatic. A magnetic resonance imaging exam was performed to exclude osteochondritis dissecans.

Comments

Marginal ossification center irregularities in the distal femoral epiphyses are extremely common in children during normal skeletal maturation, showing a high rate of bilaterality. There are four different knee ossification variants: puzzle piece (completely filled by bone), partial puzzle piece (partially filled by bone), spiculated configuration with an irregular subchondral bone plate, and extra ossification centers within the non-ossified physeal cartilage that remain separated from the condyle's ossified part. These variants may occur in the posterior aspect of the maturing femoral condyle. A subchondral bone plate focal defect results if the variant is embedded within the epiphysis' already ossified part.

Often the irregularities take a form roentgenographically indistinguishable from osteochondritis dissecans (OCD). OCD is an acquired, potentially reversible subchondral bone disorder that can secondarily affect the overlying articular cartilage and, in some cases, may lead to cartilage separation and fragmentation. The typical symptoms are pain, swelling, stiffness, locking, and clicking. Accessory ossification centers, on the other hand, do not cause any clinical symptoms and do not require treatment.

Magnetic resonance imaging provides several helpful key points distinguishing normal ossification variants from stage I OCD. Features of normal variants are infero-central defect location in the posterior femoral condyles with intact overlying articular cartilage, the presence of accessory ossification centers, lesion angle measurement <105°, spiculations, residual physeal cartilage, and lack of joint effusion and bone marrow edema. Osteochondritis dissecans MRI features have been discussed in Chap. 4 (Case 4.6).

Radiological Findings

Right knee sagittal T1-weighted MRI (Fig. 5.12) demonstrates an OCD-like lesion (arrow) in the femoral condyle's posterolateral aspect. A corresponding sagittal fat-suppressed T2 (Fig. 5.13) view shows a normal overlying articular cartilage and lack of bone marrow edema.

A left knee coronal T2-weighted sequence (Fig. 5.14) shows a posterolateral femoral condyle irregularity (arrow). Sagittal fat-suppressed fast spin-echo T2-weighted MR image (Fig. 5.15) demonstrates the normal knee maturation anatomy: heterogeneous signal intensity (SI) of non-ossified posterior femoral condyle (long arrow), hyperintense signal of organized articular cartilage (short arrow), and relative hypointense signal in the less organized hyaline cartilage of the non-ossified epiphysis.

Case 5.5: Lateral Discoid Meniscus with Incidental Fibrous Cortical Defect

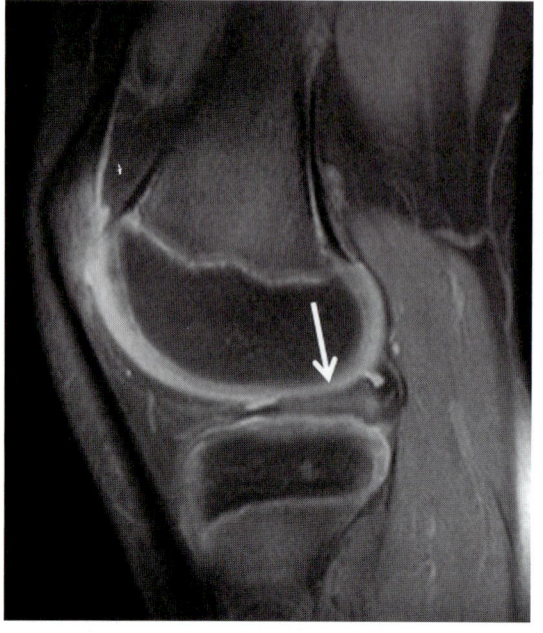

Fig. 5.16

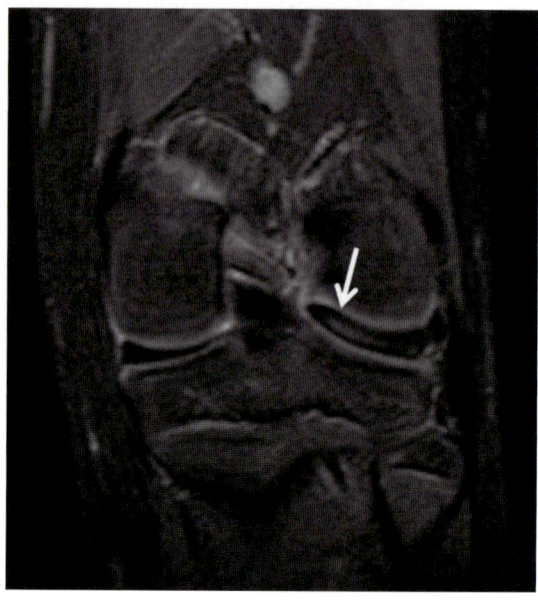

Fig. 5.17

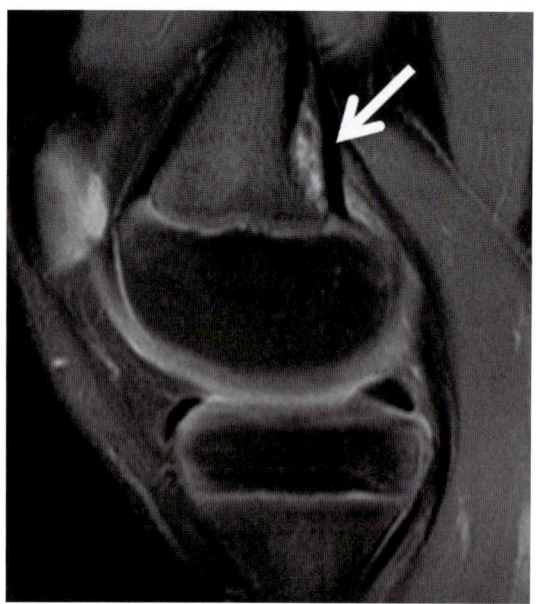

Fig. 5.18

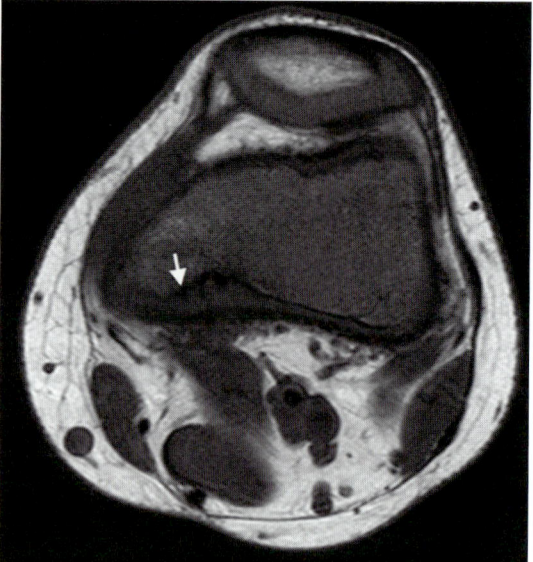

Fig. 5.19

An 8-year-old girl basketball player presented with chronic knee pain more intense while playing, with the sensation of blocking occasionally. No traumatic history was reported. At physical examination, a lateral meniscal tear was suspected.

Comments

A discoid lateral meniscus (DLM) is a common variant of normal meniscal morphology, which is usually C shaped. The enlarged body of the meniscus extends medially toward the intercondylar notch and covers the articular surface of the tibial plateau, considering three types of DLM in arthroscopy: complete, incomplete (50–80 % of coverage), and the Wrisberg variant (complete or incomplete with no capsular attachments). Their prevalence is between 0.4 and 17 % depending on the authors. It occurs on the lateral side of the knee in about 1–3 % of the population and even less commonly on the medial side of the knee. It is bilateral in up to 20 % of cases.

Magnetic resonance imaging (MRI) provides a precise identification of the lesion. According to Silverman et al., criteria for adult knees are the presence of three or more 5-mm thick contiguous sagittal images showing continuity of the anterior, and posterior horns of the meniscus are suggestive for a discoid lateral meniscus. In children, particularly those younger than 10 years should be used a ratio of lateral tibiofemoral joint space coverage. If the meniscus occupies greater than 50 % of the lateral tibiofemoral joint space, a discoid lateral meniscus should be considered. Unlike adults, children frequently present symptoms: projection on bending the knee, pain, and reduction in the range of movement. The discoid meniscus is more susceptible than normal to mechanical forces due to its thickness, hypermobility, poor vascularization, and a weak attachment of the posterior area to the capsule.

Surgical treatment is necessary in symptomatic cases, with satisfactory results following arthroscopic partial resection.

Radiological Findings

Sagittal fat-suppressed T2-weighted image and coronal STIR image (Figs. 5.16 and 5.17) show an abnormally large and thick lateral meniscus (arrow) with internal increased signal due to mucinous degeneration. The abnormal signal does not reach the articular surface (Fig. 5.17). Coronal STIR (Fig. 5.17) also demonstrates the body of the lateral meniscus extending into the intercondylar notch, consistent with complete discoid meniscus. Note the normal shape and size of the medial meniscus. Incidental fibrous cortical defect is seen on the medial condyle with hyperintense signal (arrow) on sagittal fat-suppressed T2-weighted image (Fig. 5.18) and hypointense on axial T1-weighted image (Fig. 5.19) outlined by a thin rim of sclerosis (arrow). Fibrous cortical defect and non-ossifying fibroma are discussed in length within Case 5.7.

Case 5.6: Sciatic Nerve Irritation Following a Hurdler's Fracture

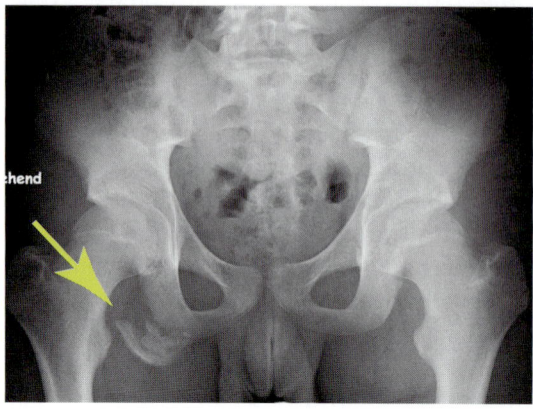

Fig. 5.20

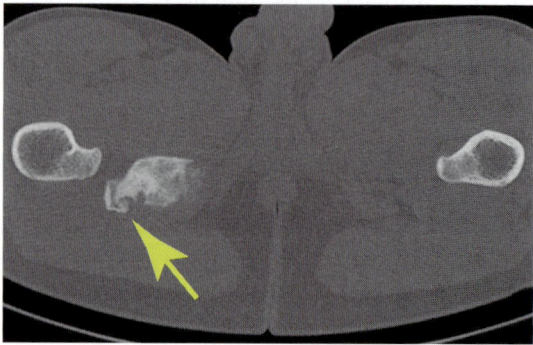

Fig. 5.21

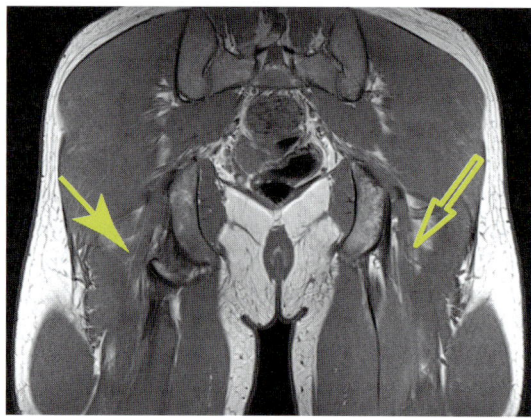

Fig. 5.22

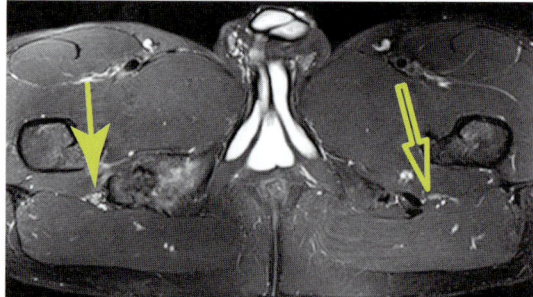

Fig. 5.23

A 16-year-old male adolescent soccer player had a grade 3 muscle injury of the hamstrings with injury of the ischial apophysis 1 year before at a soccer game that was treated conservatively. Now he complained of right electrifying and shooting pain sensations within the right thigh for several weeks, which occur when he is playing soccer but also when he is remaining seated.

Comments

Avulsion fractures of the ischial tuberosity are rare and more common in skeletally immature patients, since injuries to the apophysis can occur at all large muscle attachments when the immature skeletal structure is overstressed. Avulsion fractures of the ischial tuberosity are often the result of a violent muscle contraction, which is usually eccentric, e.g., caused by a typical "split"-like accident leading in general to sudden severe pain in the buttock with localized tenderness in the region of the ischial tuberosity. Rarely, avulsion fractures of the ischial tuberosity present in combination with sciatic nerve irritation and even late sciatic nerve palsy has been reported.

Plain radiographs, including comparison views, can usually identify the injury if the fragment is visible. Luckily, the periosteum and surrounding fascia often limit severe displacement. Surgical fixation may be considered if the fragment is of sufficient size to contain hardware, and the displacement is 15 mm or greater in physically active patients, but avulsion fractures of the ischial tuberosity are more often managed nonoperatively, especially in patients with displacement of less than 15 mm. An early diagnosis established using dedicated imaging is critical for proper treatment since prompt and intensive treatment and complete healing of these injuries are crucial in avoiding development into a potentially chronic inflammation of the muscle insertion and other late complications as presented here.

The 16-year-old male adolescent soccer player presented here suffered from a grade 3 muscle injury one year before with detachment of the hamstrings on the ischial tuberosity, i.e., ischial tuberosity fracture or "hurdler's fracture." These massive ossifying lesions have often been difficult to distinguish from infections or neoplasms, especially when these injuries occur in adults and there is not a clear history of trauma. In our case, the CT better shows the extent and anatomy of displaced bone fragment than the plain radiograph and argues against infection or neoplasm. But MRI should be used in these cases as second-line imaging technique after the radiograph for visualizing a potential irritation of the sciatic nerve and for fully assessing the soft tissues adjacent to the ischial tuberosity and the avulsed bone fragment. MRI is a highly sensitive technique as an indicator of nerve irritation by demonstrating increased signal intensity of the nerve on fat-suppressed T2-weighted images and an enlargement of the nerve as diagnostic criteria. MR imaging is a unique technique to detect the presence of nerve irritation and in contrast to electrodiagnostic testing, and dedicated neurologic examination can epict the localization of the nerve distress or entrapment and in determining its extent. Other pelvic nerve entrapment syndromes are the ilioinguinal nerve and the obturator nerve entrapment syndrome.

Radiological Findings

Radiography of the pelvis (Fig. 5.20) shows a large avulsed fragment from the ischium (arrow). The axial CT scan (Fig. 5.21) shows the osseous protuberance in direction to the sciatic nerve (arrow). 3-T MRI proves the irritation of the sciatic nerve. Coronal T1-weighted sequence (Fig. 5.22) shows the lateral displacement of the right sciatic nerve (arrow) by the avulsed osseous fragment serving as a hypomochlion – compared with the uneventful and straight course of the left sciatic nerve (open arrow). Axial T2-weighted fat-suppressed MR (Fig. 5.23) shows the increased signal intensity of the right sciatic nerve which is a sign of irritation (arrow). Also, the nerve is swollen compare with the normal signal intensity and diameter of the left sciatic nerve (open arrow).

Case 5.7: Meniscal Bucket-Handle Tear with Incidental Non-ossifying Fibroma

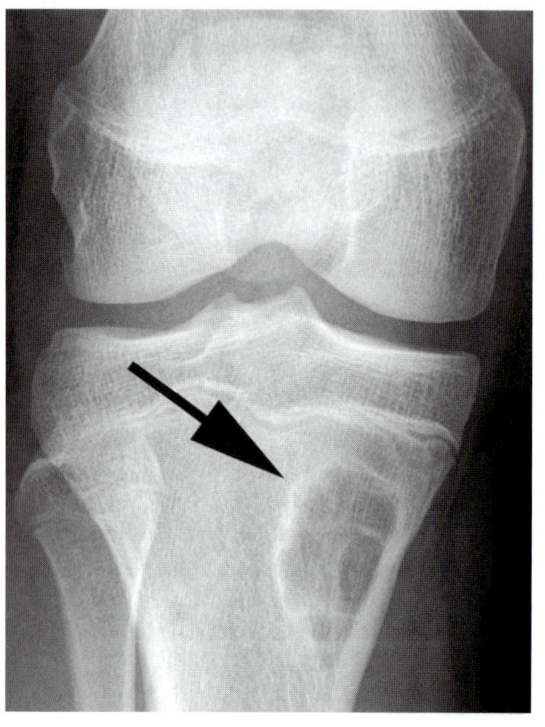

Fig. 5.24

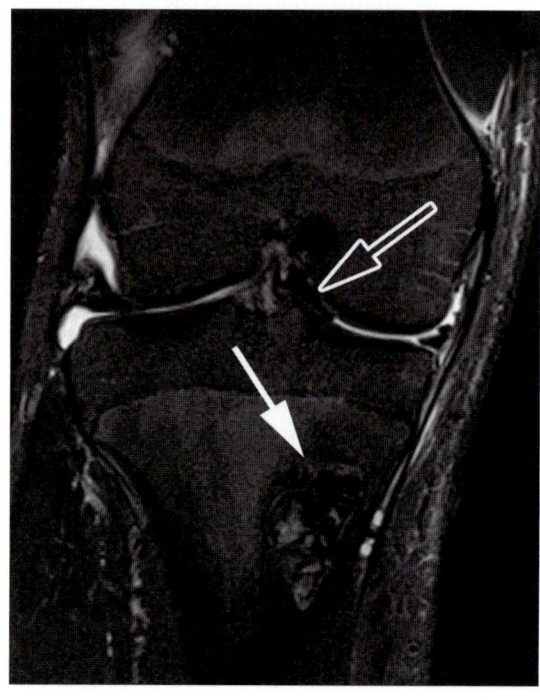

Fig. 5.25

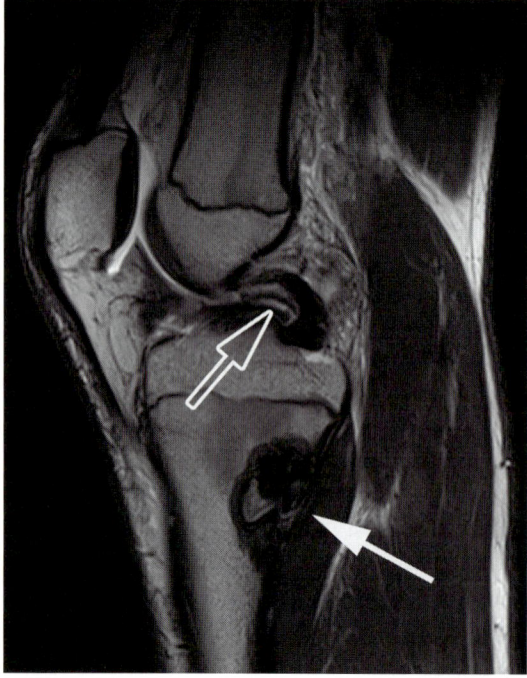

Fig. 5.26

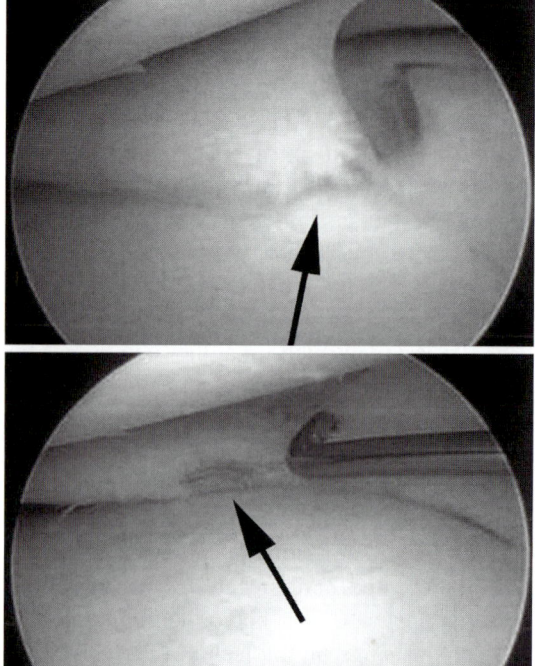

Fig. 5.27

A 17-year-old male adolescent had a distortion of the right knee when playing soccer with immediate stabbing pain, so that he could not return to play. At clinical examination, there was tenderness at the medial tibial head and no hint of joint effusion or ligament injury.

Comments

In non-ossifying fibroma, the patient age is typically less than 20 years with a male-to-female ratio of 2:1. Non-ossifying fibromas are seen on radiographs of nearly 50 % of asymptomatic boys and 20 % of girls over the age of 2 years and are commonly found in long tubular bones, particularly the tibia (43 %) and femur (38 %). Thus, these lesions are commonly encountered in the diagnostic workup of sports injuries in children and adolescents. Pathologic fractures are rare and they usually do not cause any pain. As important remark, in our case the bone lesion does not explain the clinical symptoms. The non-ossifying fibroma consists of a well-defined, lytic lesion with a sclerotic rim and metaphyseal or metadiaphysis location close to the growth plate and an eccentric, i.e., more cortical, epicenter (Lodwick 1A lesion). Non-ossifying fibromas are more likely to involve the posterior or medial cortices, such as in our case. With growth and remodelling, the lesions can be seen to "migrate" into the diaphysis and usually subsequently fill in with fibro-osseous ingrowth, becoming radiopaque when involuting in adulthood. The lesions are typically referred to as fibrous cortical defects if less than 2–3 cm in diameter and confined to the cortex. Over time, fibrous cortical defects or non-ossifying fibromas may enlarge, become smaller, become sclerotic, or disappear altogether. When the lesions become large, they appear expansile and multiloculated. The margins are typically well defined with a scalloped or serpentine configuration as a soap bubble appearance. Normally no associated soft-tissue mass or periosteal reaction is present, which in turn should prompt further evaluation to exclude a more aggressive tumor. An important notion is that when these findings are noted in a child or young adult, the radiographic appearance is diagnostic. Thus, a non-ossifying fibroma is a classic leave-me-alone or don't touch lesion. Therefore, in general no follow-up or additional imaging is necessary. The MRI appearance of a non-ossifying

fibroma is somewhat variable. Although they are essentially always low signal on T1-weighted MRI, they can have high or low signal on T2-weighted MRI. Non-ossifying fibromas have partly homogeneous or partly non-homogeneous contrast media enhancement.

Meniscal tears with displaced meniscal fragments are severe complications following knee distortions. Early detection is essential so that arthroscopic surgical repair as standard of care for patients 18 years or younger with unstable meniscal tears can be performed. Complex tears and rim width 3 mm or greater are negative prognostic factors for the clinically successful repair of an isolated meniscal tear in this age group. The typical double posterior cruciate ligament (PCL) sign has a high specificity for a displaced bucket-handle tear of the medial meniscus.

The take-home message of this case is that the incidental finding of a non-ossifying fibroma has not explained the clinical symptoms, and thus additional imaging should be performed, such as MRI.

Radiological Findings

Radiography of the knee in anterior-posterior view (Fig. 5.24), requested to rule out a tibial fracture, shows an eccentric lytic lesion with sclerotic border at the tibial metaphysis (arrow). The 3-tesla MRI examination requested by the emergency physician for further diagnostic workup of the bone lesion clearly shows that the eccentric, metaphyseal lesion (arrows) of the proximal tibia has no adjacent soft-tissue or bone marrow edema and a narrow zone of transition with no penetration of the tibial cortex. As explanation of the clinical symptoms, the tear of the medial meniscus and the medially displaced fragment (open arrow) can be nicely appreciated on the coronal short-tau inversion recovery sequence (Fig. 5.25). The sagittal T2-weighted sequence (Fig. 5.26) shows the double PCL sign (open arrow). The arthroscopic images show the meniscal tear (arrow) before (top row of Fig. 5.27) and after surgical repair by suturing (bottom row of Fig. 5.27) (arthroscopic images courtesy of Dr. Alexander Barié, Sports Orthopedics, Department of Orthopedics, Trauma Surgery and Spinal Cord Injury Center, University Hospital Heidelberg/Germany).

Case 5.8: Anterior Cruciate Ligament Rupture with Incidental Tripartite Patella

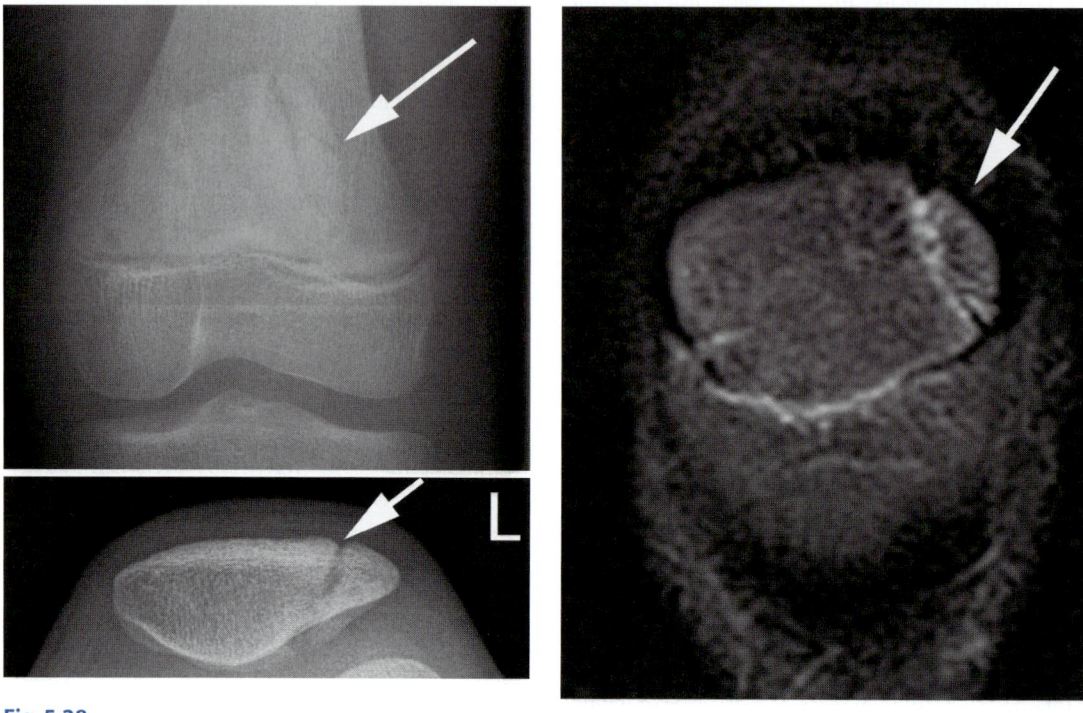

Fig. 5.28

Fig. 5.29

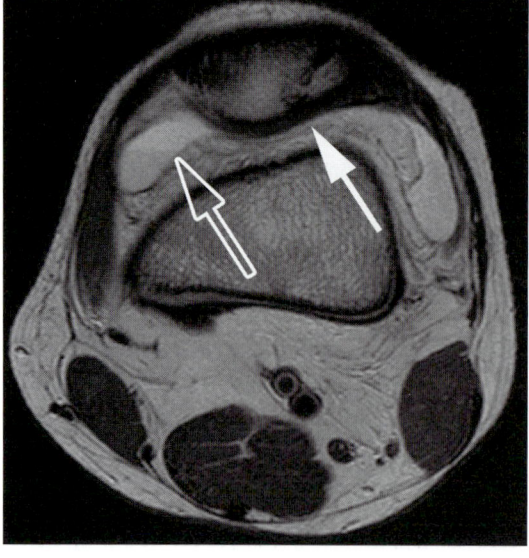

Fig. 5.30

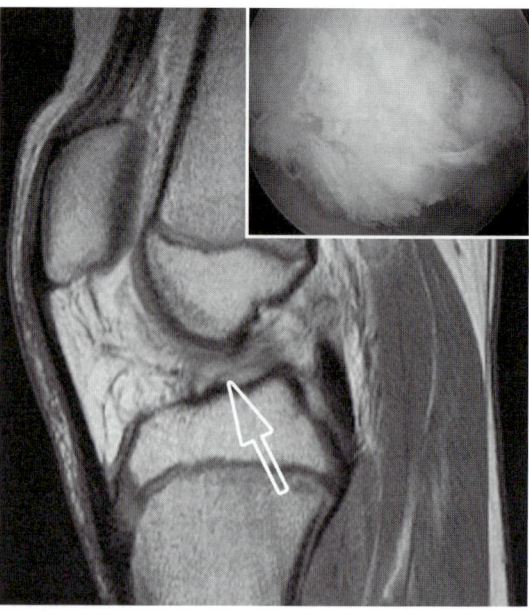

Fig. 5.31

A 12-year-old boy suffered a knee distortion at trampoline jumping. The clinical examination at the emergency room revealed only slight tenderness on palpation over the patella and no joint effusion. MRI was performed 9 days later when distinct joint effusion was clinically evident.

Comments

Normal variants of the knee are frequently encountered, and knowledge of normal anatomy as well as recognition of variant anatomy allows for a reliable diagnosis and therefore avoids misdiagnosis and over-investigation, especially in the preoperative setting. Bipartite patella is a common radiological finding observed in about 2 % of individuals and is nine times more common in boys than in girls. The term refers to a secondary ossification center that fails to unite with the main body of the patella. It is bilateral in approximately 40 % of patients. The bipartite patella may persist into adult life. This variant is typically located at the superolateral pole of the patella and is readily detected using all imaging modalities, such as in our case. Three different types of bipartite patella have been described, based on the position of the bone fragment: type I, inferior patella pole; type II, lateral margin; and the most common, type III, superolateral pole. Although usually an asymptomatic incidental finding, it may sometimes be associated with localized anterior knee pain, and then MRI is the modality of choice. In symptomatic (bi- or multi-) partite patella, MRI reveals edema and fluid at the interface of the bone fragment and native patella. On MRI, the presence of intact hyaline cartilage overlying the defect helps to differentiate this variant from a patellar fracture. Much less frequently encountered than bipartite patella, there may be more than one accessory ossification center, qualifying for the term tripartite, such as in our case or multipartite patella.

The incidence of pediatric anterior cruciate ligament (ACL) injuries is increasing in recent years. The normal ACL is composed of two bundles named for their tibial attachment, i.e., anteromedial (which is dominant in knee flexion) and posterolateral (which is most active in knee extension). Partial ACL tears can involve one or both bundles. MRI is the mainstay of diagnosis. The ACL in children normally appears thin or quite attenuated, while visibly thickening and edema suggest a recent tear. Thus, in children a thin and appropriately oriented ligament without edema is likely intact. Importantly, about half of ACL tears in young patients are accompanied by other injuries, such as bony contusions and meniscal or ligament tears.

Radiological Findings

Radiography of the left knee in anterior-posterior projection (upper row) and patella axial view (lower row in Fig. 5.28) shows a tripartite patella located at the superolateral pole of the patella with two additional patellar fragments (arrows). The coronal STIR MR image (Fig. 5.29) shows no edema within or adjacent to the ossification centers and the native patella (arrow); also the axial T2-weighted MR image (Fig. 5.30) demonstrates the intact articular cartilage overlying the defect (arrow). Note the fluid-fluid level due to hemarthrosis (open arrow in Fig. 5.30). The sagittal proton density-weighted MR image (Fig. 5.31) shows the ACL tear at midsubstance with some intact fibers near the tibial attachment (open arrow). The arthroscopic image (inset in Fig. 5.31) shows the stump of the completely torn ACL (arthroscopic image courtesy of Dr. Alexander Barié, Sports Orthopedics, Department of Orthopedics, Trauma Surgery and Spinal Cord Injury Center, University Hospital Heidelberg/ Germany).

Case 5.9: Pigmented Villonodular Synovitis

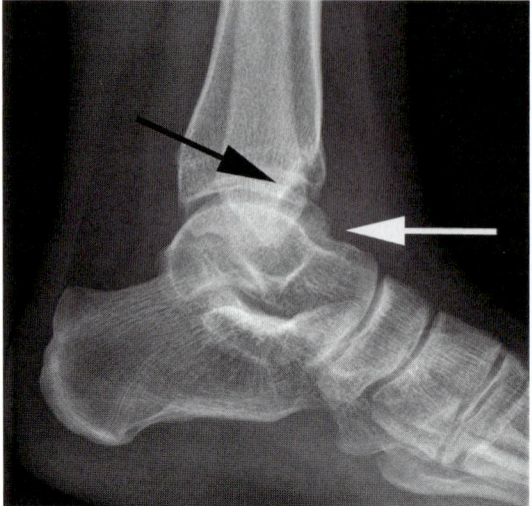

Fig. 5.32

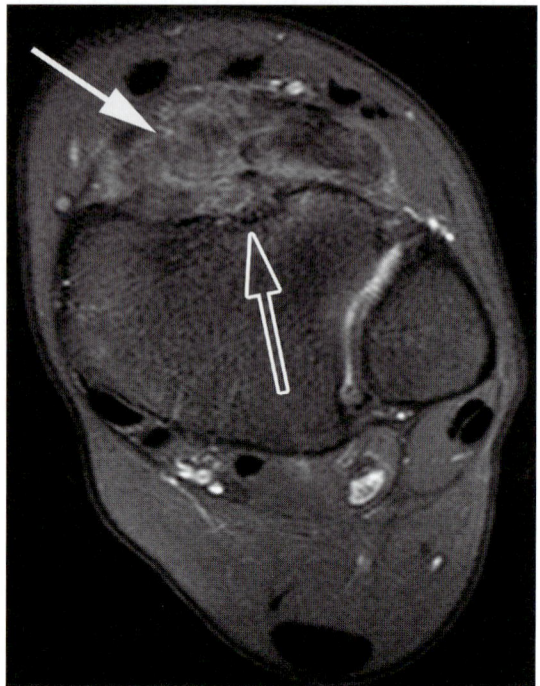

Fig. 5.33

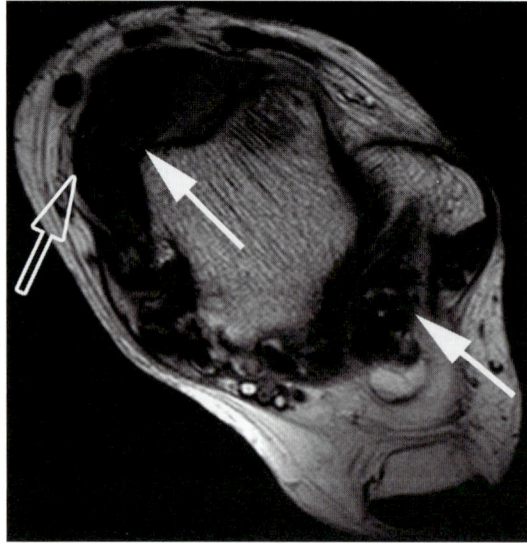

Fig. 5.34

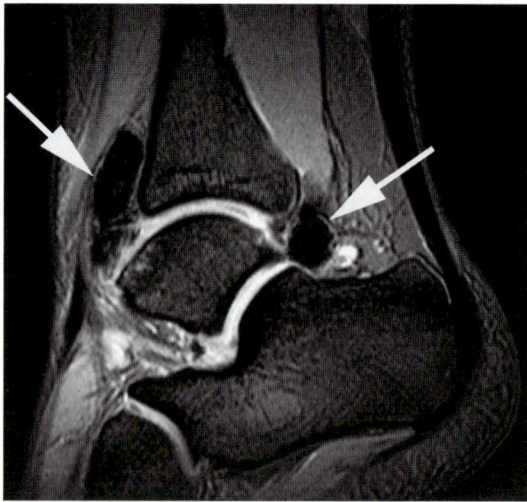

Fig. 5.35

A 16-year-old female adolescent reported about pain and slight swelling of her left ankle following prolonged sports activities for about 8 months.

Comments

Pigmented villonodular synovitis (PVNS) is relatively uncommon but potential disabling disease, which is almost invariably monoarticular. PVNS occurs in young adults (mean age 33 ± 13 years, 58 % female), mainly in the knee (75 %) but also the hip (6–16 %) and ankle joint (16 %). Patients with this condition typically present with symptoms of mild discomfort and associated stiffness of the involved joint; however, the spectrum of presentations is broad, and clinical presentation includes most often joint pain (80 %) and joint effusion (79 %) with hemarthrosis (75 %). The disorder results in increased idiopathic proliferation of synovium causing villous and/or nodular formations of synovial-lined joints. Also, it may occur extra-articularly in bursae (pigmented villonodular bursitis) or tendon sheaths (pigmented villonodular tenosynovitis). The disease can be localized or diffuse. Pathologic specimens of the hypertrophic synovium may appear villous, nodular, or villonodular, and hemosiderin deposition, often prominent, is seen in most cases. Histopathology shows multinucleated giant cells and foam cells laden with hemosiderin deposits.

Diagnosis of PVNS can be clinically difficult, and plain radiographs are usually nonspecific but may show extrinsic bony erosions with a rim of sclerosis, a finding that is most frequent with intra-articular involvement of the hip. If erosions of bone are seen, non-ossified synovial chondromatosis is a differential diagnosis. MRI is a highly diagnostic modality in characterizing PVNS when it contains hemosiderin deposits lining the synovium and exhibiting low- to intermediate-signal intensity on T1- and low-signal intensity on T2-weighted MR sequences, especially T2*-weighted gradient-echo sequences. Additionally, proliferative synovitis and/or nodules with gadolinium contrast uptake are frequent features. Thus, MRI is the modality of choice by demonstrating the distribution of the prominent low-signal-appearing PVNS masses seen with T2 weighting and the "blooming" artifact from the hemosiderin seen with gradient-echo sequences, which are nearly pathognomonic of PVNS, and by evaluating the lesion extent.

Typical symptoms of PVNS about the ankle joint are persistent pain and swelling in the lateral ankle. However, in patients who were athletically active before, their initial clinical symptoms were indistinguishable from commonly associated pathologies with persistent lateral ankle pain (e.g., tenosynovitis, osteochondral defects, os trigonum injury, and tendon tears). First-line therapy is surgical synovectomy, performed by arthroscopy and/or arthrotomy. The majority of athletically active patients can return to sports activity within a period of 12 months. The main cause of inability to return to sports is PVNS recurrence. Of note, relapse is more common in diffuse intra-articular disease due to the difficulty of complete resection, in particular with diffuse knee PVNS (30 % in one large cohort with a mean delay before relapse of 2.6 years).

Radiological Findings

Radiography of the left ankle in lateral projection (Fig. 5.32) shows an erosion of the anterior distal tibia and the neck of the talus (arrows). The axial fat-suppressed, contrast-enhanced T1-weighted MR sequence (Fig. 5.33) shows the osseous erosion (open arrow) of the distal tibia by moderately contrast-enhancing soft tissue (arrow). The soft-tissue mass has low-signal intensity (arrow) on the axial T2-weighted MR image (Fig. 5.34). Note the very low-signal hemosiderin lining parts of the thickened synovium (open arrow), which is further decreased on the sagittal T2*-weighted MR image (Fig. 5.35); these findings are characteristic of PVNS.

Case 5.10: Posterior Ankle Impingement and Anterior Talofibular Ligament Rupture

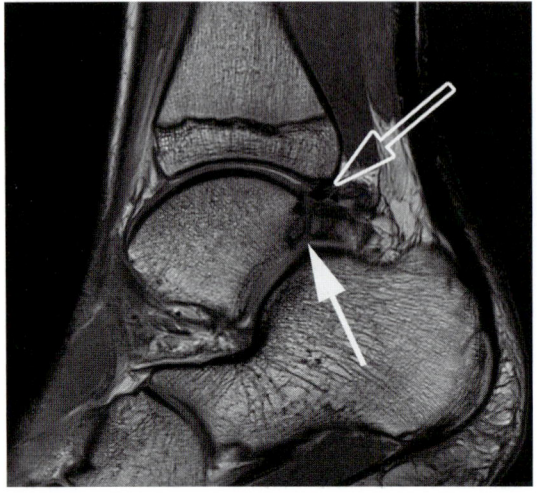

Fig. 5.36

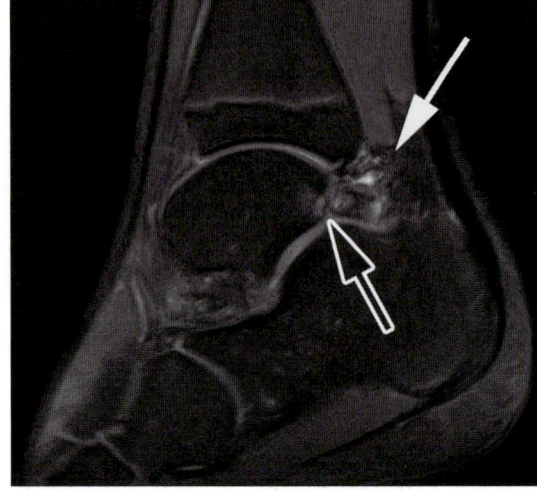

Fig. 5.37

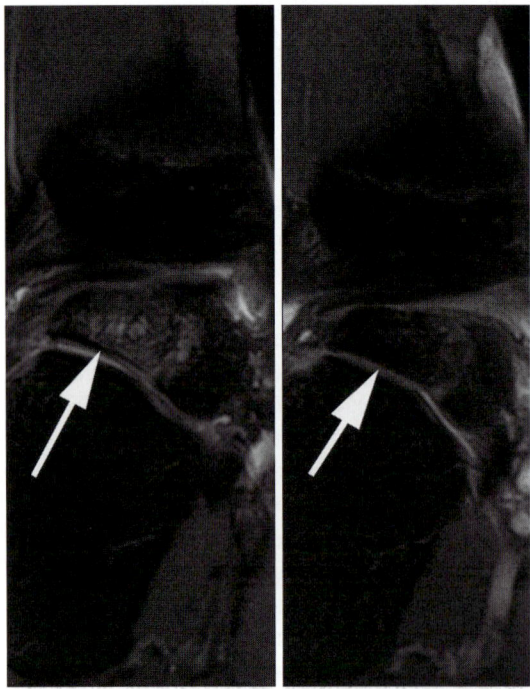

Fig. 5.38

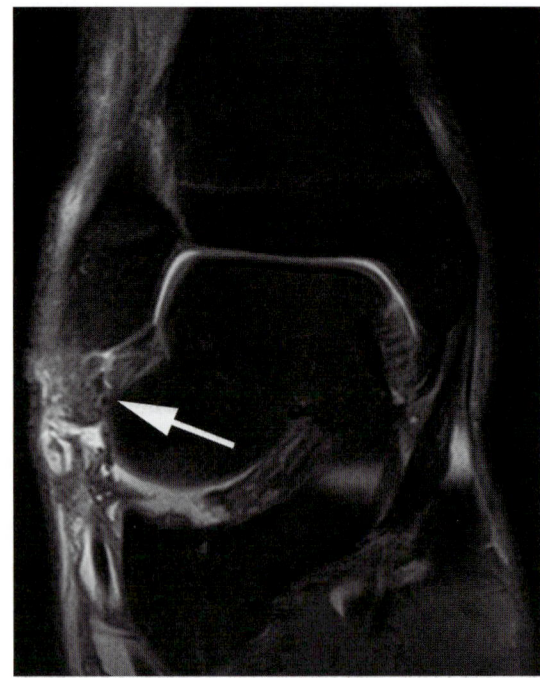

Fig. 5.39

A 15-year-old male soccer player reported about posterior right-sided ankle pain at the games and intensified training sessions, especially during sprinting and while kicking the ball.

Comments

Sports ankle injuries are mostly inversion and plantar flexion injuries that lead to damage of the lateral ligament complex with the anterior talofibular ligament as main ligament of concern. Whether the clinical stress test is positive, stress radiography can be performed to exclude a fracture. Clinical assessment is usually adequate to initially assess the severity of ligament damage, but for the evaluation of acute ankle injuries in high-performance athletes, magnetic resonance imaging (MRI) has developed to be the most important imaging procedure when the diagnosis remains clinically uncertain or when projection radiographs or ultrasound has been nondiagnostic.

Ankle impingement syndromes are classified according to their anatomical relationship to the tibiotalar joint, and they are an important cause of chronic ankle pain in young athletes, especially those who are exposed to repetitive forced plantar flexion, for instance, ballet dancers. Acute or repetitive compression of the posterior structures of the ankle (either osseous and/or soft-tissue components) can lead to posterior ankle impingement (PAI), and MRI is the preferred imaging technique for the PAI syndrome. Variations in posterior talar anatomy, such as the presence of an enlarged os trigonum or a Stieda process, i.e., an unusually elongated posterior lateral process of the talus, are the principal predisposing factors in PAI syndrome. The principal soft-tissue structures involved in PAI syndrome are the posterior ankle ligaments, the synovium, and the flexor hallucis longus tendon. PAI syndrome is common in soccer players, such as in our case, due to repetitive forced plantar flexion during sprinting and kicking the football with compression of the posterior talar process. Clinical signs are tenderness on deep palpation posterolaterally to the

ankle joint and a positive posterior impingement test with pain at forced hyperplantar flexion induced by the examiner. The MRI protocol should include a fat-suppressed T2 proton density-weighted sequence in sagittal orientation, and the ankle should be imaged in three planes. In PAI syndrome, MRI demonstrates a characteristic pattern of osseous and soft-tissue changes with the following findings often encountered together: bone marrow edema within the os trigonum/lateral posterior process of the talus and the posterior body of the talus, synovitis with distension of the posterior recess of the tibiotalar joint, flexor hallucis longus tenosynovitis, and thickened posterior intermalleolar ligament. Most patients with PAI syndrome respond to conservative treatment consisting of rest and physiotherapy.

Radiological Findings

The sagittal proton density-weighted 3-T MRI (Fig. 5.36) of the right ankle shows a large os trigonum with signs of synchondritis between the os trigonum and the posterior talus (arrow). Also, note the thickened intermalleolar ligament (open arrow). The sagittal fat-saturated proton density MR image (Fig. 5.37) better demonstrates the posterior synovitis (arrow) and the bone marrow edema in the posterior talus and the os trigonum (open arrow); the latter is also well visualized (arrow) on the coronal fat-saturated proton density-weighted MRI (left inset in Fig. 5.38). Under conservative treatment, the patient could return to play soccer, and the follow-up MRI performed 22 weeks later and 2 days after an ankle sprain injury during a soccer game revealed absent bone marrow edema within the os trigonum (arrow) in the coronal proton density-weighted sequence (right inset in Fig. 5.38). But MRI (Fig. 5.39) demonstrated soft-tissue swelling over the lateral malleolus and rupture of the anterior talofibular ligament (arrow on the coronal fat-saturated proton density-weighted sequence).

Further Reading

Books

Greenspan A (2000) Orthopedic radiology: a practical approach, 3rd edn. Lippincott Williams & Wilkins, Philadelphia, PA

Helms CA (2005) Fundamentals of skeletal radiology. Saunders (W.B.) Co Ltd, Philadelphia, PA

Keats TE, Anderson MW (2012). Atlas of normal roentgen variants that may simulate disease, 9th edn. Saunders (W.B) Co Ltd, Philadelphia, PA

Manaster BJ, May DA, Disler DG (2006) Musculoskeletal imaging: the requisites (requisites in radiology). Mosby-Yearbook Inc, Sant Louis

Resnik D, Niwayama G (2002) Diagnosis of bone and joint disorders. vol 1–5. Saunders, Philadelphia, PA

Websites

http://chorus.rad.mcw.edu/index/6.html
http://emedicine.medscape.com/article/389590-overview
http://www.gentili.net/
http://www.orthop.washington.edu/
http://www.rad.washington.edu/mskbook

Articles

Al-Hadithy N, Dodds AL, Akhtar KS, Gupte CM (2013) Current concepts of the management of anterior cruciate ligament injuries in children. Bone Joint J 95-B:1562–1569

Anderson K, Strickland SM, Warren R (2001) Hip and groin injuries in athletes. Am J Sports Med 29:521–533

Chhabra A, Chalian M, Soldatos T, Andreisek G, Faridian-Aragh N, Williams E, Belzberg AJ, Carrino JA (2012) 3-T high-resolution MR neurography of sciatic neuropathy. AJR Am J Roentgenol 198:W357–W364. doi:10.2214/AJR.11.6981

Donovan A, Rosenberg ZS (2010) MRI of ankle and lateral hindfoot impingement syndromes. AJR Am J Roentgenol 195:595–604

Earhart C, Patel DB, White EA, Gottsegen CJ, Forrester DM, Matcuk GR Jr (2013) Transient lateral patellar dislocation: review of imaging findings, patellofemoral anatomy, and treatment options. Emerg Radiol 20(1):11–23

Ecklund K, Jaramillo D (2001) Imaging of growth disturbance in children. Radiol Clin North Am 39(4):823–841

Elias DA, White LM, Fithian DC (2002) Acute lateral patellar dislocation at MR imaging: injury patterns of medial patellar soft-tissue restraints and osteochondral injuries of the inferomedial patella. Radiology 225(3):736–743

Gebarski K, Hernandez RJ (2005) Stage-I osteochondritis dissecans versus normal variants of ossification in the knee in children. Pediatr Radiol 35(9):880–886

Jaramillo D, Treves ST, Kasser JR, Harper M, Sundel R, Laor T (1995) Osteomyelitis and septic arthritis in children: appropriate use of imaging to guide treatment. AJR Am J Roentgenol 165(2):399–403

Jaremko JL, Guenther ZD, Jans LB, Macmahon PJ (2013) Spectrum of injuries associated with paediatric ACL tears: an MRI pictorial review. Insights Imaging 4:273–285

Jung JY, Choi SH, Ahn JH, Lee SA (2013) MRI findings with arthroscopic correlation for tear of discoid lateral meniscus: comparison between children and adults. Acta Radiol. [Epub ahead of print]. PubMed PMID: 23463861

Laor T, Jaramillo D (2009) MR imaging insights into skeletal maturation: what is normal? Radiology 250(1):28–38

Levine SM, Lambiase RE, Petchprapa CN (2003) Cortical lesions of the tibia: characteristic appearances at conventional radiography. Radiographics 23:157–177

Murphey MD, Rhee JH, Lewis RB, Fanburg-Smith JC, Flemming DJ, Walker EA (2008) Pigmented villonodular synovitis: radiologic-pathologic correlation. Radiographics 28:1493–1518

Paravastu SC, Regi JM, Turner DR, Gaines PA (2012) A contemporary review of cystic adventitial disease. Vasc Endovascular Surg 46(1):5–14

Rosenberg ZS, Beltran J, Bencardino JT (2000) From the RSNA Refresher Courses. Radiological Society of North America. MR imaging of the ankle and foot. Radiographics 20 Spec No:S153–S179

Santiago RC, Gimenez CR, McCarthy K (2003) Imaging of osteomyelitis and musculoskeletal soft tissue infections: current concepts. Rheum Dis Clin North Am 29(1):89–109

Saxena A, Perez H (2004) Pigmented villonodular synovitis about the ankle: a review of the literature and presentation in 10 athletic patients. Foot Ankle Int 25:819–826

Schmit P, Glorion C (2004) Osteomyelitis in infants and children. Eur Radiol 14(Suppl 4(0938–7994)):L44–L54

Thapa MM, Chaturvedi A, Iyer RS, Darling SE, Khanna PC, Ishak G, Chew FS (2012) MRI of pediatric patients: part 2, normal variants and abnormalities of the knee. AJR Am J Roentgenol 198(5):W456–W465. doi: 10.2214/AJR.10.7317. Review. Erratum in: Iyer RS (2012) AJR Am J Roentgenol ;199(1):237 [added]

Tyler P, Datir A, Saifuddin A (2010) Magnetic resonance imaging of anatomical variations in the knee. Part 2: miscellaneous. Skeletal Radiol 39:1175–1186

Venkatanarasimha N, Kamath A, Mukherjee K, Kamath S (2009) Potential pitfalls of a double PCL sign. Skeletal Radiol 38:735–779

Vilanova JC, Barceló J, Capdevila A, Dolz JL, Villalón M (2003) Angio-RM en el sistema osteomuscular. Radiologia 19:204–209

Weber MA, Rehnitz C, Ott H, Streich N (2013) Groin pain in athletes. Fortschr Röntgenstr 185:1139–1148

Zaidi A, Babyn P, Astori I, White L, Doria A, Cole W (2006) MRI of traumatic patellar dislocation in children. Pediatr Radiol 36(11):1163–1170

Printing and Binding: Stürtz GmbH, Würzburg